Praise for *Depression Fallout*

"This is a wonderful book. I've recommended it to many people who are trying to love and live with someone with depression—a truly difficult task. Sheffield is a terrific writer, her style is easy and engaging, and she has a wealth of practical advice to offer. Her stories of people who've talked to her about this problem are sure to strike a chord in the reader. She is addressing a very serious problem, because people with depression will often do everything they can to alienate those who love them, thus adding more guilt and more trouble to their already out-of-control lives."

—RICHARD O'CONNOR, PH.D., AUTHOR OF
*UNDOING DEPRESSION*

Praise for *How You Can Survive When They're Depressed*

"[This is] an extraordinary book, full of the insights that come from the fact that Anne herself was a victim of depression fallout. . . . She's got it right, and believe me, she'll help you cope."

—FROM THE FOREWORD BY MIKE WALLACE

"Anne Sheffield has guided me to fresh recognitions of myself in relation to my long-term spouse, again and again. I wish we'd had this book decades ago."

—ROSE STYRON

"Written in an engaging, articulate style, *How You Can Survive When They're Depressed* combines the personal with the practical and will serve as a gift to the millions of people who accompany the people they love on the journey to hell and back."

—MARTHA MANNING, AUTHOR OF
*THE COMMON THREAD*

## Praise for *Sorrow's Web*

"Offers important help to depressed mothers. . . . She has beautifully and eloquently captured recent advances in the study of depression and provides vital practical advice for both sufferers and those around them."

—WILLIAM BEARDSLEE, M.D., GARDNER MONKS PROFESSOR
OF CHILD PSYCHIATRY, HARVARD MEDICAL SCHOOL

"A remarkable book based on careful research. Going beyond simple 'feel good' solutions, *Sorrow's Web*'s message is skillfully couched in elegant prose and poignant personal history. Highly recommended for depressed parents, child 'survivors,' and professionals alike."

—PETER S. JENSEN, M.D., DIRECTOR, CENTER FOR THE ADVANCEMENT
OF CHILDREN'S MENTAL HEALTH, COLUMBIA UNIVERSITY

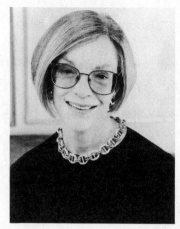

Alec Harrison

## About the Author

Anne Sheffield is the author of two well-received books on depression: *How You Can Survive When They're Depressed,* which won a Books for a Better Life Award as well as the 1999 Ken Award from the New York City affiliate of the National Alliance for the Mentally Ill, and *Sorrow's Web,* about maternal depression and its effects on children. She has worked as a scientist at the Population and Development Program of the Battelle Memorial Institute and has run her own consulting firm. She lives in New York City.

Also by Anne Sheffield

*How You Can Survive When They're Depressed:*
*Living and Coping with Depression Fallout*

*Sorrow's Web: Overcoming the Legacy*
*of Maternal Depression*

# Depression Fallout

## THE IMPACT OF DEPRESSION ON COUPLES AND WHAT YOU CAN DO TO PRESERVE THE BOND

## ANNE SHEFFIELD

HARPER

NEW YORK · LONDON · TORONTO · SYDNEY

All names have been changed to protect the privacy of individuals who have contributed to this book.

DEPRESSION FALLOUT. Copyright © 2003 by Anne Sheffield. All rights reserved. Printed in the United States of America. No part of this book may be used or reproduced in any manner whatsoever without written permission except in the case of brief quotations embodied in critical articles and reviews. For information address HarperCollins Publishers 195 Broadway, New York, NY 10007.

HarperCollins books may be purchased for educational, business, or sales promotional use. For information, please e-mail the Special Markets Department at SPsales@harpercollions.com.

FIRST EDITION

*Designed by Nancy Singer Olaguera*

Library of Congress Cataloging-in-Publication Data

Sheffield, Anne.
    Depression fallout : the impact of depression on couples and what you can do to preserve the bond / Anne Sheffield—1st ed.
        p. cm.
    Includes bibliographical references and index.
    ISBN 0-06-000934-9
    1. Depression, Mental—Popular works. 2. Love—Psychological aspects—Popular works. 3. Depressed persons—Family relationships—Popular works. 4. Interpersonal relations—Popular works. I. Title.

RC537 .S484 2003
616.85'27—dc21                                              2002069845

17 18 19 ❖/RRD 20

*To the wise and wonderful men and women who have shared their experiences on the www.depressionfallout.com Message Board*

# CONTENTS

# INTRODUCTION

Back in the days when my own depression was secretly in the ascendant, I fell in love not once but many times. Having married for the wrong reasons—principally to put as much distance as possible between myself and my mother by choosing a London-based Englishman—I returned home a few years later and embraced the role of divorced parent with a great job and a flourishing social life. Because so many members of my family had had multiple marriages, I was in no hurry to emulate them by going to the altar again, but I longed for the imagined stability of a mutually adoring relationship with the man of my dreams. As each new prospect hove onto the horizon, I enthusiastically identified him as The One. Sooner rather than later, his failings as a partner would surface, followed by ugly quarrels and tempestuous partings. In my mind, the fault lay always with him, never with me. He didn't understand me. He didn't appreciate me. He didn't do enough to make me happy or show that he cared. He just went about everything the wrong way and I was the hapless victim of his insensitivity. Nothing happened incrementally; my changes of heart were immediate and melodramatic. Despite the fact that many of my friendships, both personal and professional, ended in similar fashion and my relationship with my wonderful daughter grew progressively worse, it took me more than twenty years to recognize that my interpretation of the dynamic at work was wrong.

The dawning of self-awareness came in spurts of understanding followed by fallow periods, as though I were mentally rereading and rewriting key chapters of my life and adding an important but previously ignored character—depression. The revised first chapter recounted the long overdue discovery that I suffered from this illness, and the return of energy and purpose that medication delivered to me. The next chronicled my mother's pre-Prozac depression and its role in our mutually miserable relationship. In another I dealt with the unpleasant realization that the tattered string connecting all those past love affairs and office imbroglios was my depression, not, as I had thought, the failings of others. And last came the hardest chapter to review and reinterpret, the one that recounted the unhappiness my long undiagnosed depression had caused my daughter and how we repaired the damage.

My journey of self-discovery might have ended with chapter one were it not for the experience of a close friend who had recently married Mike Wallace of television's *60 Minutes*. Mary, an intensely private person rarely given to discussing her private life, surprised me one day by admitting to growing distress at an abrupt and inexplicable change in her previously adoring husband's demeanor. Criticism had replaced compliments. Everything she did or said was judged harshly and found lacking. What seemed acceptable to Mike one minute was deemed unacceptable the next, as though his normally logical mind had become a teetering seesaw. Whenever Mary attempted to clear the air by asking what was wrong, her questions were met with the tight-lipped assertion that nothing was the matter and nothing had changed. Over time, Mary's self-esteem dwindled. Indeed, she had come to believe that Mike's criticism of her was justified, that she was a dull, thoughtless, and unsupportive partner, but even as she accepted blame for the relationship's problems, she had grown increasingly resentful of Mike's critical assessment of her.

Loyalty and love cut the conversation short, but before closing the door on the subject Mary added one last comment that resonated uneasily in my mind: "No matter how hard I try, nothing I do is right; it's never enough, and everything always seems to be my fault," she wearily told me. "That's exactly how my mother always made me feel," I replied, and suddenly, like pieces of a kaleidoscopic pattern, the stubborn resentment and anger I still bore my mother twenty years after her death, and the feelings of inadequacy and imperfection that her endless dissatisfaction and withholding of love had engendered in me, shifted into a strange new pattern. Other telling clues flew into place: the three husbands who had loved but left my mother; the abiding dissatisfaction with her lot in life and particularly with me, her only child; the drinking; the attempted suicide; her propensity to blame everything on others, never on herself. When I added to this mix the fact that depression often travels from one generation to another, I at last had the correct explanation for my mother's behavior: She had suffered from one of the most powerful of all relationship destroyers, unrecognized and untreated depression.

The underlying cause of Mary's unhappiness finally emerged when Mike let down the barrier of silence and shared his own unhappiness with a couple of longtime friends—humorist Art Buchwald and novelist William Styron—both of whom suffered from recurring bouts of depression that had caused similar problems in their own marriages. Overcoming the typical "What me, depressed? No way!" reaction voiced by Mike, they managed to persuade him that like it or not, he was a fellow sufferer. In time, with his depression under control through effective treatment and his marriage back on track, Mike put aside concerns that his reputation as a powerhouse reporter would take a hit and decided to go public about his illness and the havoc it had caused in his work and at home. His message was unequivocably honest: "There is no way properly to describe the anguish that a depressive can put his family through. Gloom, doom, no love, no real communication, short temper, and leave-me-alone fault-finding. Why more marriages don't break up under those desolate circumstances is a puzzle, for you know deep down the damage you're doing to the ones you care about, the ones who have to live through it with you, and yet you feel somehow incapable of doing anything to lighten the burden." This act of personal courage, sustained in speeches to audiences throughout the country, has brought Mike Wallace deserved acclaim and the gratitude of millions of Americans who battle daily with a depression they strive to hide from others. Mary Wallace, overcoming her natural reticence, has joined her husband in spreading the message that depression is a family affair. Together they have encouraged many depression sufferers to seek treatment; a far greater number are either unaware of what ails them or fearful of the stigma enshrouding it.

The similarities between Mary's experiences and mine suggested to me that the presence of depression adversely affects relationships and has a predictable emotional impact on non-depressed intimates. To satisfy my curiosity, I began tentatively sounding out others whom I suspected of loving someone with a depressive illness and found two in my immediate circle of friends. They needed little encouragement to talk; a brief recounting of my recent epiphany was all that was needed for them to unlock carefully guarded gates and for the first time allow their hurt and distress to come pouring out. Not only did their experiences closely mirror mine, but both used many of the same phrases to describe their feelings as though all of us were reading from some universal script. By now persuaded that depression fallout might be a widespread phenomenon, I started attending a weekly support group for friends and family of someone suffering from depression or manic depression. There I discovered that all the members of the group, whether parent, child, spouse, or lover, were traveling through the same five overlapping stages that constitute the symptoms of depression fallout: confusion, self-blame, demoralization, resentment and anger, and, finally, the desire to escape the source of so much unhappiness.

What had begun as a journey of self-discovery became

a book, *How You Can Survive When They're Depressed: Living and Coping with Depression Fallout.* The book in turn spawned a Web site, www.depressionfallout.com, set up for me by a computer-whiz friend of my daughter's, who suggested that it would help promote sales and, through links to other Web sites concerning depression, be of value to those who wished to learn more about this illness. Internet dodo that I was back then, I failed to note that the opening page of the Web site invited viewers to click on a message board. Although I had billed the book as a surrogate support group for depression fallout sufferers deprived of this luxury, the concept of broadcasting information usually reserved for close friends and psychotherapists was so foreign to me that I never thought to click on the message board and investigate what might be there. When I finally did four months later, I was stunned to discover that the Board, with zero input on my part, had become a flourishing cyber-support group. And far from my hazy notion that only bored teenagers with screen names like Force One, Beachbum, and Dingbat Woman hang out together on the Internet, I found a fellowship of thoughtful, civil, depression fallout sufferers who were willing to share their personal experiences in detail, quick to respond supportively to those of others, and interested in learning everything they could about depressive illness. The overwhelming majority of those posting were married to or in a long-term relationship with a partner suffering from depression or manic depression.

Shortly after my delayed entry onto the screen, the one-thousandth message was posted. Since then, the numbers have grown exponentially, with some one hundred stalwart posters in crisis at any given time. Messages headed "Help me put this in perspective, please!" and "My depressed husband's 'reality'—how do I cope?" ring familiar fallout themes that resonate with fellow sufferers and draw supportive and helpful replies. There is always a troupe of so-called lurkers waiting on the sidelines, who read silently for weeks or months before gaining courage to write their opening messages: "I am losing the love of my life," "End of rope," "Scared and confused." Once categorized as "oldies" or "newbies," all come to think of themselves as "doobies," as in, "I do be having problems with this depressed person in my life." On the Board, familiarity breeds not contempt but cyber-friendship and solidarity. When Ginger's mother underwent cancer surgery, she turned to her fellow posters for a shoulder to lean on; when Phil's father died, he received loving wishes and sympathetic support. Everyone knows that depression fallout is draining and renders one ill equipped to deal with crisis.

I have come to understand that the anonymity provided by the Internet is a great leveler. Racial and ethnic differences, sexual preferences, and top or bottom economic and social backgrounds have little bearing on the problem at hand. What counts is whether or not you are a depression fallout sufferer. As in any support group, many whose problems have been resolved eventually fade away. Recent arrivals benefit from the wealth of past posts, yet each has a new twist, a previously unvoiced question to ask, another insight or bit of wisdom to offer. What attracts newcomers and also keeps so many oldtimers coming back is the comfort of commonality induced by the details offered:

- The list Jill made to guide her behavior while waiting for her depressed husband's medication to kick in— sympathetic understanding, no nagging about helping with the kids, no bitchiness in response to his being mean, no joining in the fights he constantly picked— only to have him announce in two weeks that he "doesn't want to be around me NOW! Why?"

- How LP's depressed boyfriend offered to return her overdue books to the library, but "the whole time he's offering to do this kind little thing for me, his eyes are just burning with anger, and yes, hatred, and his body language is stiff and tense beyond belief."

- Purple's account of a hopeful heart-to-heart talk with her husband during which he acknowledges that something may be wrong with him but rejects the possibility of depression, and Phil's wistful reply, "This is only from a pathetic guy-type perspective but it sounds pretty good to me. He told you he loves you, he said he doesn't want to lose you or his daughter, and that he wants to try harder to work things out. I'd give a lot to hear even just a little bit of that kind of talk from my depressed wife."

- Jay's admission that he had cried during a downer scene with his depressed wife, and a flow of supportive admissions from other posters, both men and women, that they "had cried a river" or "done buckets of the stuff," and that crying is natural and necessary to grieve. "Most people should probably cry more to let themselves 'feel' their feelings," echoed another fallout spouse, "something I know my husband is too 'macho' to do."

As posters read the minutiae of exchanges between other couples and of the reactions they provoke, they soon begin to note how similar their own experiences are. What had seemed an isolated nightmare is suddenly perceived as a widely shared problem: "For the first time in my life I have found other people who know what it is like to walk this road." "This Board has made me realize that I am not a bad person for having certain feelings." "You guys have helped me be more compassionate and even-keeled at home." "I'm so glad I found this group as you have given me the strength and courage I've needed to get through this." "Thanks to coming here, I don't feel guilty about my anger anymore. Seems like it's a normal reaction under the circumstances."

The Message Board users are a tightly knit but widely dispersed family whose members live throughout the United States and overseas as well. Some are construction workers or secretaries; some are engineers, teachers, small business owners, or corporate managers; one is a missionary. They range in age from seventeen to seventy, live in big cities and small rural towns, and encompass both the hard-pressed financially and the owners of summer homes. Having little bearing on depression fallout, these superficial differences evaporate. Some posters are living with a depressed partner in denial, some with a spouse or lover tentatively trying a first medication, and an unlucky few have suffered with their mate through suicide attempts and hospitalizations. Others are contemplating separation or divorce, but as you will discover, or perhaps already have, writing "The End" to a fallout story is seldom simple.

Once I had belatedly cottoned to the Board's thriving existence, I checked it regularly but rarely posted myself except to suggest that advice seekers refer back to this or that section of *How You Can Survive When They're Depressed* for answers to their questions—until one post zapped my authorly pride. "Most of us here are being left by our undiagnosed depressed partners, if not physically, then emotionally," the poster observed, "so I wonder why Anne's book says it's only 'cured' depressed spouses who leave?" The answer is that the Board's collective experience in this instance, and in some others as well, runs counter to the prevailing views of many psychiatrists and psychotherapists whose research informed my first book. It became increasingly clear to me that the posters knew more about this problem than the experts, and that they were posing questions for which neither the professionals nor I had ready answers.

Lively exchanges about other situations scantily covered or ignored in the first book sprang up: What do you do about the other man or woman who often figures prominently in ongoing Board sagas? What's "fair" behavior when you are dealing with a disagreeable and recalcitrant depressed person? Why do many depressed people become addicted to Internet porn sites? How do you know when suicide talk is manipulative behavior and when it's for real? What can you do about alcohol abuse when your depressed person won't listen to the pdoc's (prescription-writing psychiatrist) advice? It became painfully obvious that the single chapter I had addressed to depression fall-out husbands, wives, and lovers was pitifully inadequate to my readers' needs. By then, thoroughly persuaded that what happens when depression enters a marriage or long-term relationship deserved a book of its own, I turned to the Message Board for confirmation. The response, imme-diate and enthusiastic, was summed up by one dedicated poster from the Board's earliest days. "I think this is a GREAT idea," wrote Gwen. "I've actually been hoping you'd come up with a notion like this, simply because I am truly impressed by the wealth of information we seem to have compiled on this board."

Therein lies the essential contribution made by the Message Board to this new book. The posters have jointly constructed an extraordinarily honest, detailed, and oth-erwise unavailable record of what happens to a relation-ship when depression sneaks in the back door. The vivid, poignant stories aren't "case book" studies from the note-books of therapists and marriage counselors; they are real-life accounts by people like yourself who have found a medium to express their troubled thoughts and feelings and exchange observations on the behavior of their depressed partners. This book distills their experiences and coping strategies, as well as those of countless others in similar situations whom I have come across in other ways, and also draws on the findings of psychologists, psychiatrists, and other mental health professionals who have made depression and interpersonal relationships the focus of their study. To this mix I have added my belated understanding that the effect of my mother's depression on me was only the first step of my own journey of self-discovery, and that all those serial, mangled relationships upon which I hopefully embarked over the years crashed and burned due to my unrecognized depression and the mindset it imposed upon me. So I am not just a purveyor of other peoples' sad tales; I provide plots of my own that mirror those told in the succeeding chapters.

Loving someone who is depressed brews confusion, frustration, resentment, and pain. Learning that your involuntary reactions are thoroughly normal is a giant first step toward regaining equilibrium. Another is provided by the array of effective coping strategies presented in this book. An unanticipated third step forward is the discovery that a sense of humor can be found even in the unpleasant depths of depression fallout. So should your hitherto devoted spouse or partner announce out of the blue that he or she has decided to leave you, not in the heat of anger but in a tone more suited to a discussion of which movie to see, compare his or her comment with the following Message Board Letterman list of the ten most frequently cited reasons for wanting to end the relationship:

10. Being with you isn't fun anymore.

9. You don't know what it's like.

8. You think I'm an alcoholic just because I drink a lot.

7. I have bad Karma and can't do anything about it.

6. You can't understand me.

5. You don't accept me for the way I am.

4. It's better this way.

3. You're not the same person I married.

2. I no longer love you, but let's stay friends.

1. I don't want to talk about it.

The Kafkaesque nature of the list is an apt introduction to the what-on-earth-is-going-on essence of depression fallout, the five stages of which are described in Chapter 1. Chapter 2 lays out the panoply of the most common depressive illnesses and their symptoms, and can be used as a rough diagnostic tool by fallout partners to check out whether their mates are indeed suffering from one (or several) of them. Depression usually endows its victims with extraordinarily efficient blinders that blot out self-awareness; when combined with the persistent stigma conveyed by the term "mental illness," the blinders work as barriers to the decision to seek treatment. Overcoming denial, the topic of Chapter 3, is an all-important barrier that non-depressed partners must hurdle if the relationship is to survive and prosper. Chapter 4 addresses the issue of setting boundaries that can limit the stress and damage caused by prototypical depressive behavior, which often warrants the label of emotional abuse.

The treatment of depression involves far more than popping pills; unless the non-depressed partner is a well-informed and active participant in treatment, the effort he or she has put into overcoming denial may be for naught. How they can learn to distinguish between good and bad practitioners and judge whether or not the proffered prescriptions for antidepressant medication and therapy are doing their job is the subject of the fifth chapter. Loving and living with a depressed person, whether or not he or she is in treatment, drains energy and self-esteem. In Chapter 6, fallout mates are encouraged to put aside the guilt most experience whenever they address their own needs and wants.

Even the most experienced and knowledgeable fallout partners are baffled by depression's apparent ability to kill their mates' capacity for love. Chapter 7 explores this enigma and its implications for the relationship's future. The decision to stay in a depression-damaged partnership and put it back together post-treatment, or to break the bond—with all the attendant considerations, including the well-being of children—is addressed in Chapter 8. The final chapter—"Life Beyond Depression Fallout"—visits with some of the Message Board posters who have opted for one or the other of these two routes and takes a look at how they are faring now. The Appendix is a guide to navigating the rich plethora of Internet resources on every aspect of depressive illness, from abstracts of professional journal articles on the latest depression research to the Web sites maintained by the leading mental health organizations in the United States and abroad.

A primary goal of this book is to convey to fallout partners the convoluted workings of the depressed psyche and its ability to warp and misinterpret reality. Early in this brief Introduction, I referred to the tardy realization, despite long-present evidence, that I had unwittingly inflicted on my daughter the same brand of fallout pain to which my mother had subjected me. It amazes me that that shattering discovery came not before but during the writing of my second book, *Sorrow's Web: Overcoming the Legacy of Maternal Depression*. What better proof could there be of the power of this illness to trick the mind and flood it with siren songs? As a sufferer of depression and of its fallout, too, my compassion extends to both camps. What separates them is the illness itself: common, treatable, and dangerous as a shark.

# Depression
# Fallout

# 1

# The Deadly Duo: Depression and Depression Fallout

Love and depression speak different languages. Every man and woman in a relationship touched by depression comes face to face with this unpleasant truth. Although each believes that he or she is living through a unique situation, the behavior of both parties conforms to a predictable pattern. One participant acts according to the dictates of his or her depression: Be critical, unpredictable, sullen, illogical, angry, touchy, put-upon, distant yet occasionally tender, and deny there is anything wrong with you. The other follows the rules governed by depression fallout: Be confused and bewildered, blame yourself for the relationship's problems, become thoroughly demoralized, then get angry and resentful, and, finally, yearn to escape.

Few people are well informed about the dynamics of depression and its companion, depression fallout, despite the unhappiness they cause. Ask most people to conjure up the image of someone who is depressed and they will envision a huddled figure sitting passively in the corner and murmuring about how sad he or she feels. No wonder, since most lists of depression's symptoms begin with "a persistent sad, 'empty,' or anxious mood," followed by "loss of interest or pleasure in ordinary activities, including sex." While these symptoms do describe how depression sufferers feel, they are not matched by the expected passive behavior. Indeed, the depressed often become unpleasantly aggressive, argumentative, and faultfinding without provocation. This disconnect causes innumerable depression-clouded relationships to unravel and become mired in conflict and misunderstanding. When previously attentive, warm, demonstrative partners turn irritable, distant, and thoughtless, mates are unlikely to attribute the change to a psychiatric illness, even though they may have read about depression in the abstract. Instead, they jump to what seem to be more likely explanations: a waning of affection, dissatisfaction with the marriage or love affair, a clandestine liaison with somebody else, a selfish preoccupation with work, or a reluctance to share deep, dark secrets that concern both partners.

Since the true culprit is an illness that afflicts no less than nineteen million Americans at any given moment, why don't depressed partners speak up and explain what is going on in their minds and hearts? Surely anyone whose life has turned inexplicably gray and hopeless would choose to talk about it with his or her intimates, thus paving the way for answers and solutions. But that is not depression's way. Indeed, depression's most insidious trait is the ease with which it seduces its sufferers into blind alleys signposted Lousy Relationship, Bad Karma, Weak Character, Stress Overload, and other misleading names.

All those battered by depression fallout are convinced that their situation is unique and their reactions to it aberrant. Having enjoyed a gratifying and seemingly solid partnership beset by no more than the usual ups and downs, they find themselves living with an unwelcome stranger masquerading behind a familiar face. Not only does this newcomer no longer behave as expected, but he or she appears to have undergone a personality change for the worse. Tenderness and support have been traded in for grumpiness and irritability; sharing for secretive distance; patience and reason for volatility and antagonism; and good habits for bad ones. Threatening though this is, fallout partners do not seek solace or advice from family and friends. Convinced that they are somehow responsible for the transformation, or that its explanation is perhaps embarrassing and best kept hidden from others, they guard their secret. This extracts a costly price.

Isolated in self-imposed solitary confinement, unable to coax explanations or apologies from their mates, fallout sufferers start shelving their lingering suspicions of personal responsibility and take to building protective ramparts in the form of negative reactions to and feelings for their partners. Loosening the knot of love, loyalty, and companionship formed over time takes a toll, and that toll is at least partially paid by fallout partners in guilty self-recriminations for being a "bad" or selfish person who can be counted on for support in good times but not in rocky ones. They indulge in tit-for-tat, parrying criticism with criticism, and although this temporarily relieves their feelings of frustration, it brings them no closer to an understanding of what is happening to the relationship.

The first gift the Message Board delivers to new arrivals is assurance that they are neither malcontents nor misfits. They quickly learn that even those Board posters whose partners have been diagnosed and are being treated for depression share the same problems and are subject to the identical negative thoughts. Even in the presence of such empathetic company, first-time Board visitors often lace their posts with "I know you won't believe this, but . . ." or "He [or she] said the strangest thing to me . . ." and are instantly welcomed and reassured that what they had thought unbelievable and strange is commonplace. When oldtimers respond like a well-rehearsed chorus—"Oh, yes, we know, we've been there, too, and we understand"—the dam of reticence gives way, allowing pent-up emotional turmoil to flow freely. In short, the single most important fact for a depression fallout sufferer to grasp and take to heart is that his or her particular brand of misery, far from being unique, is shared by a minimum of nineteen million others in the United States alone, and so are their far-from-aberrant emotional reactions.

## THE HAVE-I-GOT-DEPRESSION-FALLOUT? QUIZ

Your initial task is to determine if this illness does have a grip on your partner, but depression is a master of disguise, capable of appearing on the scene without any tell-tale rashes, coughs, or fever. All you are sure of right now is that your good relationship is coming unglued for no identifiable reason and that your partner is behaving in strikingly unfamiliar and unpleasant ways. Rather than asking if he or she might be depressed, which probably will be countered by outraged denial, do some detective work on your own state of mind. Start by reading the following similes composed by Board posters who rose to the occasion when asked to complete the sentence, "Trying to have a relationship with a depressed person is like . . .

- playing one huge game. The problem is, it's a game for which it's difficult to come up with a winning strategy. Nothing logical, as in other games, works. The depressive [posters refuse to use the politically correct "depressed person"] seems to know what keeps you in the game and uses that against you. It's a long, scary, sad game because it involves someone you love and you hate to see the person become your opponent."

- being on a roller coaster blindfolded."

- trying to unlock your car with a long, spindly coat-hanger wire. It seems like if you could just . . . get . . . the little hook . . . on the door lock you could . . . it would be so easy if just . . . oh . . . I think I have it . . . DRAT! . . . Count to ten, breathe, breathe, don't smash the window . . . breathe . . . okay, start again . . . move the hanger . . . almost there. . . ."

- banging your head against a brick wall. It takes you a while to figure out that you need to put your helmet on, and even then it still hurts."

- walking across a floor strewn with marbles. You're doing just fine, kind of keeping your balance, but working really hard at it, when all of a sudden— WHAM! No matter how many times you try, you end up on your butt."

- picking your way across a minefield because a child is crying on the other side. You have to do it or you would never forgive yourself, so you tiptoe gingerly on, each step bringing you to fuller realization of the hazards. Every now and again your foot touches something and your heart stops and you freeze, thinking that this may be the time everything explodes. Onlookers see only a field of poppies and cornflowers, so they're wondering what the hell your problem is. To them, it all looks idyllic, peaceful, and calm; to you it's an inescapable nightmare."

If several of the above elicited a "That's just how I feel!" reaction, rate yourself a possible depression fallout victim (and your partner a possible depression sufferer) and continue the test. Next, chart the ups and downs of your emotions since you first realized that an indefinable something sent the relationship off its normal track, and see if you can accurately place yourself in one of the five overlapping stages of depression fallout.

If you inhabit its initial stage, confusion, you are in a

state of shocked bewilderment induced by a seeming change for the worse in the person you fell in love with. You are probably wondering why the endearing qualities that attracted you to your mate in the first place seem to have gone into hibernation. Instead of the warmth and affection to which you are accustomed, he or she has withdrawn, become cool and distant. Where once they were communicative and sharing, they now are disinclined to talk, not only about the distance that has developed between you but also about work, the kids, plans for the weekend or vacations, or the myriad topics you used to gab about routinely and that cemented your bond of intimacy. They used to be decisive and exercised good judgment, qualities you prized and relied upon, but now they change their mind and mood so often that you feel tentative and insecure. Gone is their sense of humor; in its place is a somber heaviness that blocks all your attempts to leaven the atmosphere. They have replaced "We" with "I," making you feel as though you are no longer part of the equation. Remarkably, even the children are subjected to the remoteness and edgy temper that characterize this strange new person in your life. Most unsettling of all, everything you have enjoyed doing together no longer holds your partner's interest. You are rejected in the bedroom, and even casual affectionate overtures, a hello kiss or a friendly tap on the shoulder, seem unwelcome.

Perhaps you have already moved on to depression fallout's second stage: self-blame. If so, you now are pretty sure that the problem is your fault. Perhaps you've been spending too much time on your job or your parenting responsibilities. Or you've let yourself go, gained some weight, stopped paying attention to your appearance, and the love of your life has strayed from your side as a result. You promise yourself that you will shift your focus from your own interests and needs to your partner's, lose ten pounds, get a great haircut, come home with flowers, reignite the premarital excitement, rejuvenate the magic between you. You dwell on all those little bones of contention that you thought so unimportant at the time: the vacation suggestion you nixed because it was too expensive, the movie you didn't want to see, the weekend sales conference you had to attend, too many hours spent at the gym, the fuss you made about the chores left undone, the night you sulked when you should have sparkled. You embark on a serious campaign of reform, planning activities you know your mate enjoys, accommodating your wishes to his or hers, giving in without arguing, and doing everything you can to become the perfect spouse or lover. But your campaign is a flop. No matter how hard you try, things between you worsen.

If you have reached stage three, demoralization, your self-esteem has hit rock bottom. Feeling graceless and inept, everything you do and say seems off-base and inappropriate, as though your center has disappeared. You allow the reality of your past history together to seep away and acknowledge that, in truth, you have little to offer as a partner, are far less wise and attractive than you had always thought, and probably as difficult to live with as your mate relentlessly insists. Assertions that you are unsupportive and a nag sound plausible. And since your energy and enthusiasm are at ground zero, and just getting through each unrewarding day is exhausting, when your partner repeatedly claims that if anyone is depressed, it is you, you find yourself in agreement. After all, isn't this exactly how depressed people are supposed to feel?

Resentment blooms in stage four. You begin fighting back, but in negative rather than positive ways. Demoralized and drained, you discover that combat is energizing, and defend yourself with spirit. Matching your own behavior to your partner's surly, irritable style, you shoot off some accusations and hurtful rejoinders of your own. The unfairness of it all sets you seething; what's going on is *not* your fault and you do *not* deserve this treatment. Since sane communication as an avenue to reconciliation and mutual understanding is no longer an option, your resentment simmers, often erupting into full-blown anger. Although sporadically exhilarating, anger cannot suppress the essential truth that you are still deeply in love with your combatant, despite the adversarial present, and long for the "real," pre-depression beloved to miraculously reappear. You feel trapped in a no-win bind, fearful that whether you push or give in, you will still lose the battle for the relationship's survival.

Sooner or later, the accumulative emotional burdens imposed by stages one through four weigh so heavily that you enter stage five: a longing to be free of unhappiness, and of the person who is its source. If that is where you are in the depression fallout journey, you are perhaps toying with a temporary separation, buying yourself time to assess the future from a distance. If your partner has already proposed one, or if he or she is spouting divorce-speak, a baffling practice of many depressed mates, the situation may seem not only intolerable but pointless, even though you still long for a reconciliation. Or perhaps you have settled into a bloodless arrangement built on psychological if not physical distance, often opted for by partners with children, and are contemplating years of cool cohabitation for their sake.

If you recognize yourself as inhabiting one or, more likely, several of the five stages outlined above, give yourself an A on the fallout quiz and consider yourself welcomed to depression fallout territory. Your mate has joined the ranks of the depressed. There is, of course, an ideal solution: Persuade your partner that depression is the root problem and that he or she needs to be treated for it, and then jointly set about the difficult task of restoring harmony and intimacy. So why is this not the usual outcome? Because those who suffer from this illness—and I am one of them—are usually unaware of what ails them until hit over the head with a sledgehammer. Even after repeated blows, most refuse to entertain even the hint of such a diagnosis and stubbornly dodge the risk of having it confirmed by a professional, whether a family doctor, psychiatrist, psychotherapist, or marriage counselor. When you and other intimates broach this reasonable step, it is angrily dismissed out of hand as not only untrue but insulting. The non-depressed find such reactions perplexing and bordering on dim-witted, but rereading the introduction of this book should remind you that depressive blindness is unrelated to intelligence.

Two statistics are relevant to the depression fallout quiz: One in every five people has been, is, or will be blindsided by depression at some point in their life, and half of all American marriages now end in divorce. While depression is far from the sole culprit in broken relationships, a growing number of experts (among them psychiatrist Peter Kramer, author of *Listening to Prozac* and *Should You Leave?*) believe that this illness is often the cause rather than the result of divorce, as previously thought. No one has ventured a guess as to how many premarital relationships meet a similar fate, but judging from both the Message Board and readers' E-mails, it is safe to say that depression separates lovers with surgical skill and is a major home-breaker. As you will learn in a later chapter, many researchers in the fields of psychology and psychiatry have taken a close look at depression-ridden partnerships and concluded that the deck is stacked against them for as long as the illness goes untreated.

When fifteen years ago a coworker suggested that I, like he, might be depressed and in need of medication, I loftily informed him that I had always been a bit moody, a condition I secretly considered indicative of an admirable sensitivity and emotional complexity. Somewhat intrigued by the prospect of chatting with the superexpert psychiatrist he offered to call on my behalf, I trotted off to my appointment fully expecting to be told that I was a fascinating exception to the rule. After an interview lasting ninety minutes, to my surprise the psychiatrist confirmed my coworker's suspicions. I caved in on the spot, relieved to know that the horrible way I felt was not my fault but

an illness, and in time my life turned right side up again.
Unfortunately, my reaction was not entirely typical. For
many men and women, the double whammy of depression
blindness and the stigma still clinging to this illness acts as
a formidable barrier to acceptance of the diagnosis.

People with depression are no more weaklings or deadbeats than are people who have heart disease, diabetes, or
cancer, yet a significant number think of themselves that
way. Even though the stigma is less potent today than in
the past, uninformed, stereotypic attitudes continue to
impede a swifter change in public opinion and personal
assessment; long established ways of thinking are hard to
break. If more family members were aware that depression's unofficial symptoms include a predilection for criticizing and blaming others, anger, a touchiness that
approaches paranoia, wishy-washy thinking, and impaired
judgment, instead of assigning them to other causes, many
depressed partners might be encouraged to acknowledge
their illness and its impact on the relationship.

If you are still unsure whether your partner's behavior
is generated by depression or by what one Board poster,
exhausted by more than a year of her husband's depressive temperament, long ascribed to an advanced case of
"jerkism," the following four stories will help clarify your
thinking.

## FALLING INTO FALLOUT

Everyone resists being pigeonholed as a typical example of
this or that. If, for instance, you just recently settled into

married life, surely your experience has nothing in common with that of a thirty-year marital veteran and mother of two grown children. Yet just a few days apart, two newcomers to the Message Board—Windswept and Ivy— provided ample evidence that a partner's depression can wreak havoc at any stage of a relationship. As you read their stories, bear in mind that gender has little bearing on depression-fueled behavior. Though depressed men and women are not identical twins, they behave toward their partners in remarkably consistent ways.

Ivy says she noticed a change in her husband right after they returned from a blissful honeymoon. He turned cold, distant, and uncommunicative. For five interminable months she kept asking what was wrong and he snapped back that nothing was wrong, he was just tired. By the time her birthday arrived, his seeming lack of love had led her to view their marriage as a mistake. The "celebration" was a horrendous bust. Although he produced a bunch of flowers, he had no card or present for her, and his lame excuse, "Too busy at the office so I never made it to the bank," did little to reassure her. He had had several beers while waiting for her to arrive and seemed unfriendly and primed for combat; the lack of a welcoming kiss was only the opening round. Every time Ivy opened her mouth to speak, her husband told her to stop interrupting and threatened to leave if she did it again. "And he did," she writes. "He stalked out and left me sitting there alone at the table. He didn't even pay. I finally asked for the check and went home. I feel as though I'm living a nightmare."

Ivy, too new at the game to realize that she was sharing

a story that will probably have a happy ending, wrapped up her post by saying that a few weeks later her husband came home from the office and blurted out that he was suffering from depression and had started taking antidepressants. Instead of relieved, she felt betrayed and shut out. "Why did he keep his illness a secret from me?" she writes. "For five months I have been thinking that something was wrong with me. He has withdrawn from me and won't even let me touch him. I don't know what to do. I am so hurt. I am in so much pain."

A Board veteran quickly sets her straight: "Yep—that's depression at work and it's tough stuff. But," she adds, "your husband has admitted to it and is taking medication without any urging from you. I know it's hard for you to realize it right now, but you're actually a lucky woman. A lot of us here are dealing with denial or refusal to get help." After suggesting that both of them bone up on depression and its treatment, she offers a basic piece of fallout wisdom: "The way he's behaving has nothing to do with you personally. Somehow this illness creates an astonishing self-centeredness and lack of empathy for others, especially loved ones. It still hurts terribly to be on the receiving end; all of us here know that." You will discover in later chapters that a dogged preoccupation with oneself, as though nobody else in the world mattered, although missing from the standard list of depression's symptoms, comes with the territory. If mistaken for a true change of heart, it will make you question your affection for your partner just as it has led him or her to do the same.

At first glance, Windswept's story sounds very different

from Ivy's. She and her husband, whom she still dearly loves, have been married for thirty years. A decade ago he was diagnosed as suffering from manic depression, an illness characterized by long periods of deep downs interspersed with out-of-control manic highs, and until recently medication prescribed by his psychiatrist had kept things on an even keel. She joined the roster of posters because her husband recently had announced out of the blue that he wanted a divorce in order to "live by himself and be free," that he has felt nothing at all for her over the last ten years, and that she has given him neither the companionship nor the support he needed and deserved. This appalling rejection has devastated Windswept. "I am so overwrought with grief that I don't know what to do. I know as much as anyone about depression and am desperately trying to see if I really have let him down to the extent he says." Yet she took part-time jobs when her husband was too depressed to work, tenderly cared for him and their children during the worst periods, grew vegetables to sell and feed the family, and, when he had his last breakdown and was hospitalized for four months, drove two hundred miles twice a week to see him. Only an expert in depression fallout will understand how she can question her attention to her husband's needs. Intensifying her pain is the upcoming wedding of their son, which, should she acquiesce to his wishes, she will attend as a divorcée.

"I miss my husband so much and he hasn't even left the house yet," she writes, spattering tears through cyberspace. "When I try to dissuade him, he says his mind is made up and the conversation turns very ugly." Like many posters, Windswept read the Board for a month before posting her own story. "Many of you have had similar experiences. How do you remain sane?" she asks. "I have invested my whole life in my family. They always came first. They mean everything to me. Need help. Need advice," she closes.

Of the many supportive replies, those from Ginger and Megan are particularly pertinent. Ginger's sheds light on a killer bomb dropped by many depressed people: "When they say they haven't loved you for however many years, or even that they have never loved you, remember that their outlook, including their perceptions about their past history, is twisted toward the negative. While there may be some truth in what they say about our faults (who among us is perfect all day every day, year after year?), they blow our shortcomings out of all proportion." My view, less temperate than Ginger's, is that sufferers of this illness find fault whether perfection exists or not; so determined are we to see ourselves as righteous and our partners in the wrong that we manage to edit our memories to suit that purpose. As to staying sane, Ginger continues, "It isn't easy but it's doable." Support, whether from family members, friends, the Message Board, a therapist, a member of the clergy, or a church group—whomever you feel you can confide in—is essential. "Don't try to cope with this without help!" This advice, in an expanded version, is important enough to merit a later chapter of its own.

Megan weighs in with her prescription for regaining equanimity. At fifty-plus she recently exited stage five and opted for a definitive split. Still shaky a year later, but optimistic and in possession of her self-esteem, she explains how she recaptured it. "Fall in love with yourself. Go back to when you were younger and find the points in your life where you glowed and felt good. Do now all the things you gave up doing to make room for being the perfect wife and mother." When Megan got divorced, she says, her grief was extraordinary, but she learned that it actually felt good to "cry and yell and yank out weeds and get down and dirty with the pain. I've come out now on the other side, the brighter, sunnier one. Time will bring you there. In the meantime, you need to keep doing ANYTHING that feels good. Give yourself at least one year for grieving and reward yourself for being alive. Be strong. Be weak. Above all, be human, and grow through this. You can and you will."

It's hard to project a rosier future while languishing in depression fallout, especially when there are children to consider. Board posters Phee and Nick each have kids to worry about, his aged two, four, and six and hers nine and eleven. Phee announces that finally, after laboring under the delusion that her husband would stop denying his depression and start living if only she could just pin him down and find the right words, she has "gotten it." Having put aside all hope of reconciliation, she is now working toward a university degree and the prospect of a salary sufficient to support a single mother of two.

Nick, his family's sole breadwinner, is not dreaming of divorce; although his wife has been depressed for half of their eight years together, his devotion to her is unwavering. Contrary to the majority of posts, Nick's contain neither hints of resentment and anger nor pleas for sympathy. All he seeks from the Message Board are some suggestions for stirring his depressed spouse into action without hurting her feelings. He packs compassion, concern, and drama into one terse paragraph that begins, "My wife is a wonderful person and mother when she's not depressed, but lately she's depressed all the time." No shirker of responsibility, Nick cleans the house before going to work, then cooks and spends the evening being a parent to compensate for the five hours per day his wife whiles away in depression chat rooms before prostrating herself in front of the television. His every attempt to air the problem, summarized as "all those things that never get done," and to arrive jointly at solutions is short-circuited by his wife's single-minded insistence that his attitude, not her depression, is to blame. "Please don't spend so much time on the Internet, you need to be there for the kids" earns him the accusation that he is trying to control her life. When he readily agrees that the friends and support she finds there are important, but adds that their three sons need support and attention, too, she claims the reason she's depressed is because he's forever telling her what to do.

Nick's message drew immediate replies, most of them focusing on the probability that the antidepressant his wife had been taking for some time was not the correct one for her. Ask if she would allow him to sit in on her next visit to the prescribing doctor, one suggested; if she refuses, another pointed out, the threat to the children's well-being in this instance justifies going over her head and calling the psychiatrist with a succinct, nonemotional report on their home life. Others recommended that he set clear boundaries to delineate what he would and would not tolerate in the way of behavior—no computer after the kids get home from school, no TV until the dinner dishes are washed—and told him to stick to them no matter how unpleasant his wife's initial reaction might be. She'll be really angry when you turn off the switch, they warn, but keep doing it, don't lose your temper or be drawn into a scene, and sooner or later the message will register. One bitter recent divorcée advised him to "get out before you lose your sanity." "I love her and I'm not giving up on her," Nick shot back. "I tell her every day I'm there for her. And I know deep down that she's really trying to cope with her depression."

Nick knows he did not cause his wife's depression, but judicious reading between the lines reveals the strength of his conviction that he has somehow failed her, that in his effort to keep the household running he has inadvertently trampled on her self-esteem and unfairly added to an already heavy burden. His version of the second stage, self-blame, illustrates depression fallout's chameleon ability to change appearance without losing potency. Rare is the fallout victim able to shut the door on one phase before jumping into the next; instead, non-depressed partners accumulate a collective burden of feelings that feed each other and pile up as the relationship deteriorates. By the time they reach the final stage of longing for escape, guilt, demoralization, resentment, and anger are all still fighting for supremacy.

Phee's energetic two-page post, introduced with an

apology for sounding like "one sarcastic lady," never mentions love. "My depressed husband's behavior is the same old same old," she writes, specifying self-centeredness, apathy, hostility, excessive use of computers, and no grasp on reality, followed by a chain of etceteras. Despite her assertion that the light has dawned at last, she admits to frequent "weak" moments when she still wishes to love and to please her husband despite knowing that it will bring no rewards. "It's lucky I'm resilient because, believe me, I don't intend to live like this forever. Even when occasionally he's being civil, he seems to consider me a poor wife. I'd be thrilled if he found one he thought was better and left me and our kids without a fight." Behind Phee's bravado is the wistful hint of a continuing attachment to her husband of thirteen years, or, more accurately, to the pre-depression person she had married and briefly rediscovered when he decided to give up smoking and was prescribed Zyban, also marketed as an antidepressant under the brand name Wellbutrin. "When his gray fog suddenly dissipated, we realized that what I called 'jerkism' was really depression, and for fourteen months everything was great again. But then he decided he was 'cured,' never mind the doctor's warning, and all hell broke out again. End of story." "Welcome to the Seriously Confused Club," the first reply begins. "What is it with depressed people? Why can't they get it? What about this crazy denial thing and what can you do to overcome it? Are we all married to the same person?"

Answers to these questions are provided in later chapters, together with an understanding of the Alice in Wonderland world into which the depressed fall. But for now, here is a simpler question: Is it possible for a new bride, a wife deserted after thirty years of marriage, a devoted father of three, and a spouse longing for divorce to undergo a similar experience? The short answer is yes. They differ only in the fallout stages each is currently straddling and in the information about depression and its treatment to which each can accurately lay claim. Windswept, Ivy, and Nick all need reminding that effective treatment for the depressed partner is the key to emerging together on what Megan calls that other, sunnier side. Since Ivy writes that her husband broke the news about his depression and medication only a few days ago, she doesn't yet know that although antidepressants work their miracle in about 60 to 70 percent of cases, there is a lag time of two to six weeks before they take effect. In the interim, Mr. Ivy is going to be broody, touchy, and thoroughly pessimistic. The idea that a little once-a-day pill is going to work some miracle seems pretty outlandish to him right now, so he anticipates a lifetime of misery. That's a hard place to be.

Windswept says she knows as much about depressive illness as anyone; thankfully, she is mistaken. Having lived with a manic-depressive husband for thirty years, she does indeed appreciate that his complex illness is hard to stabilize and keep under control, but she may be unaware of recent advances in its treatment. Some cases of depression that appear hopeless to average practitioners are solved by the superexperts, whose research keeps expanding the treatment universe. Since the only psychiatric facility within striking distance of Windswept's home is in a rural area and not connected to a teaching hospital, it is perhaps unable to attract cutting-edge physicians skilled in fine-tuning a mix of medications.

Early depression fallout sufferers—Ivy is a good example, as was Phee before Zyban caused her husband's gray fog to evaporate—pay their dues in stages one and two: confusion and self-blame. None are spared stage three, but those few who are exceptionally resilient, as Phee claims to be, manage to hoist themselves more rapidly out of demoralization and switch on the resentment and anger of stage four. Windswept's stubborn devotion to her husband, unshaken by his outrageous behavior and rejection, glues her to stage three yet fails to shield her from resentment. How long she endures their combined tyranny will depend on her tolerance for mistreatment and, I suspect, on the long shot that a superexpert will come to her, and her tormented husband's, rescue. Nick's place on the fallout continuum is harder to discern. My guess is that he is designing his own version of demoralization, one that still retains features of the same self-blame that once sparked Phee's hope of eventually finding the right words or actions to blow her husband's denial to smithereens. But to do that, Nick will have to help his wife find, if not a psychiatric star, at the least a more competent psychiatrist.

What happens in the fifth and final stage, a wrenching longing to free oneself from the morass of frustration and unhappiness, depends in part on factors beyond one's control, such as the timing and severity of the illness. Resilience and a capacity for stress, qualities that appear to be the products of willpower, actually originate in one's genes. One must also acknowledge the specific circumstances that have defined the relationship's history: the strength of the bond, the quality of communication between both partners before depression appeared, its impact on children and on family finances, the presence or absence of emotional support available to fallout sufferers, and a host of other variables.

Even if they are currently stretched, bonds long in the making can take a lot of pressure without snapping. Jay, a resilient fallout survivor hovering at the doorstep of escape, says that his depressed wife had become a "thoughtless, mean, uncommunicative, and unloving woman." His post describes a joint therapy session during which Jay admitted that there were days when he wanted to stay married, and others when he didn't, and that it was increasingly hard for him to go on trying to save the relationship when he had no idea what his wife wanted and she made no matching efforts. Jay then openly aired his suspicion that his wife wanted him to suggest divorcing so she couldn't be accused of being the "bad guy." Asked by the therapist if that was the truth, his wife agreed, but added that giving up would be an admission of failure on her part. Jay's interpretation of that statement, shared by other posters who had engaged in similarly surreal dialogues, was that "the only way my wife fails is if she didn't work hard enough at saving our marriage. That means, once again, that everything wrong needs to be *my* fault. I have to take the blame for us falling apart despite her 'best efforts,' just as I have been asked to take the blame for everything else that goes

awry. It's never my wife's fault, she never accepts blame for
our problems," Jay moans. But even fallout stories that
seem fated to end in separation or divorce can take an
unexpected upturn. As of today, Jay and his wife, whose
psychiatrist found the right antidepressant for her on the
third try, are still together and working toward reparation
rather than separation.

Not all stage-five citizens have good news to share.
Janice, whose husband has been seeing another woman,
warns readers of her message's content by heading it "Too
good to be true. A very long story." Her impassioned post
pours out the news of his extramarital affair, his admission
of guilt, his promise that it was only a "misguided fling,"
his fervent claim that he still loved Janice and was committed to their marriage, and then his lapse from grace,
not once, but twice. Throughout, her husband repudiated
the physician's diagnosis of depression and refused treatment. This couple did divorce; Janice did the untying, is
happy with her decision, and has moved herself and her
kids back to her hometown, where she is teaching school
and successfully rebuilding her life.

Most of stage-five territory is occupied by spouses and
lovers unsure of what they want. Typical of many of them,
Jams is terrified that her lover of six years will decide to
leave. The night before her first posting, she had tried to
have a conversation with him, but he dismissed her feelings, "basically acting as though nothing had happened
and that things should go on as normal, meaning he
ignores me and does whatever he wants." This time, says
Jams, she did not chase after her husband to apologize and

beg him to treat her better. She is still deeply in love and doesn't want him to leave, but her mind and her heart are tugging in opposing directions. "I want him to stay with me and work on getting well. But if he is not willing to try to get well and is going to go on treating me so badly, I know the best thing for me is to be away from him so that I can heal enough to feel like a person again. I'm so sure that he's going to tell me he doesn't know what he wants, and that it will be best for him to leave. That's going to hurt like hell, but I have to look after myself and move on, right? How do I convince my heart of that?"

If you, too, are mired in emotional turmoil, suggesting that you now turn your attention to a lesson on the interplay of genetics and the environment and how they affect the brain's neurotransmitters to induce depressive illness may sound like a waste of time. It isn't. The more you know about this illness, the better equipped you will be to deal with its entry into your life via the person you love. You will find the following chapter far more gripping than expected, especially since it includes not only depression science but also some revealing thoughts and comments from a number of people just like your depressed husband, wife, or lover.

# 2

# Unraveling the Mind-Brain Mysteries of Depression

The ubiquitous use of "I'm so depressed" to describe distress about everything from a waistband that no longer buttons to the forecast of rain for the weekend reinforces the misconception that depression is a passing mood best dealt with by pulling up one's socks and taking a brisk walk. In novelist William Styron's memoir of his own experience of depression, he says that when he first became aware that he had been undermined by this illness, he felt a "need to register a strong protest against the word *depression*," even when used accurately. Pointing out that it used to be termed "melancholia," a word in English usage for some seven hundred years, he noted that it has now been "usurped by a noun with a bland tonality and lacking any magisterial presence, used indifferently to describe an economic decline or a rut in the ground, a true wimp of a word for such a major illness."

By any name, depression is a biological illness so serious that the World Health Organization and the World Bank rate it as a leading cause of disability in the United States and worldwide, and the American Medical Association considers it the most incapacitating of all chronic conditions in terms of social functioning. In 1997 its annual cost to society was $43 billion, a staggering sum representing the combined costs of two hundred million days lost from work, poor performance on the job, psychotherapeutic care, and the loss of lifetime earnings due to suicide. Some 15 percent of the men, women, and children caught in its despairing grip end their own lives. Although depression is also closely correlated with heart disease, diabetes, stroke, cancer, and other serious illnesses, and although the number of those afflicted appears to be steadily rising, this potential killer is consistently underrated by the general public and often undetected by health professionals.

When you ask your depressed person what's wrong and receive the usual reply, "Nothing," rest assured that an army of experts is proving him or her wrong. Scientists from multiple disciplines long separated by methodological and conceptual differences—among them neuroanatomy and neurophysiology, pharmacology, molecular and cellular biology, genetics, and the cognitive and behavioral sciences—now work closely with psychiatrists and psychologists to zero in on the precise mechanisms involved. Diligence, technology, and a few serendipitous "Eureka's" hold out the promise of even more effective, and side effect–free, antidepressants. In the meantime, push past your partner's unwelcoming rejoinder and deliver today's good news: The currently available antidepressant medications and adjunctive treatments can pull approximately 80 percent of depression sufferers out of their personal hellholes.

If depression heralded its arrival with itchy red spots, swollen glands, a high temperature, or a hacking cough, the world would be a happier place. Instead, minuscule changes throughout the brain, undetectable by current diagnostic tests, are made manifest in the mind. In the absence of obvious physical clues, depression and fallout sufferers alike are tricked into blaming shifts in thinking and behavior on erroneous culprits such as boredom, dissatisfaction, and the need for a change, but the truth is that when the brain is impaired, so are the emotions. A well brain "instructs" the mind to respond to a lottery win with elation; a brain malfunctioning due to depression transmits the message that the lottery officials have made a mistake, quite probably for the express purpose of raising, then dashing, dreams of glory. Recognition of the immutable connection between mind and brain, so baffling to the layperson, is aiding scientists in their search for better understanding, but depression remains one of the great unsolved medical mysteries.

Topflight researchers readily admit that depressive illness, despite exhilarating advances over the last decade, remains a difficult puzzle to assemble. Each new piece of information that fits neatly into place puts others in question and requires reassessment of previous findings. Surprisingly little is known about the grapefruit-sized bundle of tissue that makes us tick. The principal reason for this is the astonishing complexity of the human brain, which contains about one hundred billion cells, or *neurons* as scientists call them. The possible interconnections or *synapses* between neurons are estimated to exceed the number of atoms in the universe. Communication between them is made possible by the *neurotransmitters,* which act as chemical messengers that jump the infinitesimal synaptic gap between cells in less than one five-thousandth of a second, generating behavior. For decades, compelling evidence pointed to the faulty functioning of three neurotransmitters—norepinephrine and dopamine (both close chemical relatives of adrenaline) and serotonin—as the cause of depression's onset. Painstaking research by some of the best scientists the world over has proven that this explanation is a simplistic view of a far more complicated, and still poorly understood, interactive mechanism.

Today's research stars are more cautious and refer to dysfunction of these neurotransmitters as only one in a cascade of dominoes that ripples through and affects multiple areas of the brain that determine how we think, feel, and behave. These specialized parts of the brain regulate appetite, thirst, sleep, and sexual desire; handle the fight-or-flight response; are responsible for how we gauge emotional reactions such as elation, excitement, anxiety, rage, and aggression; and modulate our capacity to start and stop behaviors associated with these emotions. Bear this domino effect in mind while reading the section on depression's symptoms, but first a word about depression's causes.

Sufferers of this illness are usually too busy trying to cope with its negative effects on their psyches and lives to wonder why they have it and their neighbors don't, but the correct explanation would dispel any suspicion that they are psychologically weak and lacking moral gumption. Majority thinking in the field implicates an inherited gene or, far more likely, a complex of genes, as the cause of depression. Since no one has actually located that gene or genes, and because the illness is more apt to appear after puberty than during childhood, chances are that what is passed along from one generation to the next is not depression but a vulnerability to it. Vulnerability may blossom into depression because it has been triggered by a stressful event such as loss of a loved one, job, income, health, or even status.

Scientists now agree that psychosocial and environmental factors also play an important role. A childhood characterized by emotional or physical abuse, or by prolonged deprivation and isolation, may lead to permanent changes in brain function that increase susceptibility to this illness. Another trigger fast gaining status is stress, because the hormonal system that regulates the body's response to both physical and psychological stress is overactive in people with depression; vulnerability to stress, like vulnerability to depression, is transmitted genetically. Some researchers tie the rising prevalence of depression to the meltdown of previously stabilizing and nurturing institutions, in particular the traditional family, and to skyrocketing drug abuse.

## GENDER DIFFERENCES IN DEPRESSION

One of the few facts about depression that has resisted serious challenge is that more women than men suffer from it, by a ratio of two to one. But this is open to controversy, as anyone willing to sit down and plow through the more recent academic studies on gender differences can see. The factors cited for the discrepancy are biological, psychological, and social. On the biology front is an as yet unproven link between the female sex hormones, reproductive events, and depression. Boys and girls have similar rates of depression until puberty, at which time it doubles in girls, equalizing after menopause. Also suggestive are male-female differences in circadian rhythm patterns. This complex system regulates sleep and activity over each twenty-four-hour period and may explain why women are more likely than men to suffer from hypersomnia (excessive sleeping) when they are depressed. Also cited are striking differences in the way men and women metabolize thyroid hormones, which are closely related to mood disorders. Psychoanalysts and feminists cling to the outmoded belief that there exist both a "feminine" personality and a "depressive" personality, and that some link exists between the two.

More interesting, and also more persuasive, is the role of social factors particular to women in today's society, including their dual work and family responsibilities, the rise in single parenting and all the burdens it entails, sexual discrimination, and a shrinking of the traditional support systems that protect women from isolation. Common sense dictates that all are contributing factors, but evaluating their precise impact on women's depression rates involves more guesses than hard answers. Here, too, there is some evidence to the contrary. When one researcher took a hard look at spousal absence, social isolation, financial difficulties, and health problems, she found that women were neither more nor less apt to develop depression symptoms than were men in the same pickle. But in this research study, as in many others, the results may have been skewed by chance selection of female participants who were more resilient than the norm.

Recently, some depression epidemiologists, who look at depression from a statistical vantage point, have postulated that women do not actually suffer from depression twice as often as men, but that the sexes have different styles when it comes to this illness. Women are thought to turn inward, becoming less active and more subjective and ruminative about the causes and implications of their depressed mood. Men, on the other hand, react to it more physically, turning outward to activities that distract them from how they feel. Anchoring this assumption is the theory that men and women have differing "pathways" to depression, the core of which is the belief that women get depressed over relationships and men about achievement-related issues. Emerging research may prove that this is yet another stereotypic shibboleth. Diane Spangler, a clinical psychologist at Brigham Young University, sampled a group of 427 male and female outpatients seeking treatment for depression and found no substantiating evidence for the pathway thesis. If she and other like-minded researchers are correct, this lets female hormones off the causal hook, thereby exploding yet another promising explanation for the two to one ratio.

## SOME VARYING PERSPECTIVES ON THE SYMPTOMS OF DEPRESSION

Whatever its cause or causes, and by whatever pathway, depression announces itself with a typical array of symptoms both physical and psychological, but how they are described and interpreted depends on who is doing the diagnosing. Doctors have a neat and tidy list of symptoms that is best described as the Detached Professional Observer's List. The one compiled by fallout sufferers reflects a day-in, day-out involvement with their partners' depression; I call theirs the Unofficial Symptoms List. Depressed people's inability to concentrate and think rationally, paired with a sense of helplessness and hopelessness, inhibits their list-making ability; nonetheless, one intrepid sufferer posted hers on the Message Board and titled it "What depression means to me." I have grouped her list, together with some heart-wrenching bulletins from other depressed partners who have visited the Board, under "Notes from the Underground" (see page 46).

### The Detached Professional Observer's List

When doctors diagnose depression, they look for what they call a "depressed affect," loosely translated as apathy and negativity, and then ask a few straightforward questions: Have there been recent changes in sleeping and eating patterns? Are you a bit more irritable or tearful than usual? Do you have more trouble concentrating and remembering things? As a rule, general practitioners steer clear of queries about their patients' private lives, so their diagnosis of depression will depend on what they can see and what they are told about the following symptoms of depression:

- a persistent sad, "empty," or anxious mood

- loss of interest or pleasure in ordinary activities, including sex

- decreased energy, fatigue, being "slowed down"

- sleep disturbances (insomnia, early-morning waking, or oversleeping)

- eating disturbances (loss of appetite and weight, or weight gain)

- difficulty concentrating, remembering, making decisions

- feelings of hopelessness, pessimism

- thoughts of death or suicide, suicide attempts

- irritability

- excessive crying

- chronic aches and pains that don't respond to treatment

The classic rule of thumb is that the first two symptoms are the preeminent indicators of depression; if one of them plus any four of the others have been present for two weeks or more, all day or most of every day, an antidepressant prescription will probably be forthcoming from the doctor.

Despite this widely published symptoms list, there remains much misunderstanding and confusion among laypeople about what does or does not qualify as depression, largely because of the variety of terms used. Those most frequently employed are clinical depression, mild or moderate depression, severe or major depression, mood disorder, and unipolar illness. Except for the qualifying adjectives indicating their severity and, therefore, their ability to disable, these are all the same illness. Some who suffer from mild, untreated depression are able to function well enough to fool the outside world for some time. More often, once the barrier of mild is crossed, depression becomes sufficiently disabling to wreak havoc at home and in the office.

The above symptoms list is a serviceable tool for clinicians, but they see only one-third of the nineteen million depressed Americans; the other two-thirds are either unaware they have the illness or choose not to admit its presence. A significant number of those who do seek a physician's help will take the medication prescribed for a week or two and pronounce it useless (effects usually take hold in four to six weeks), or will discontinue it due to side effects (which can range from loss of libido to dry mouth and constipation, depending on the drug and individualized reactions to it). Others will take the medication sporadically (there will be little or no improvement), or quit as soon as they feel better (the depression has a fifty-fifty chance of returning).

Not all physicians are infallible. Many otherwise competent general practitioners fail to give proper credence to a patient's symptoms and miss the diagnosis entirely, while others minimize the seriousness of the illness. Patients may be treated to the bootstraps prescription. Suggestions to get away for a while, find a new challenge or hobby, exercise more and eat better are followed by well meaning instructions to "get rid of all that stress you're under." This is all fine advice, but no match for depression. Doctors may order expensive and worrisome tests to determine the cause of recurrent headaches, backaches, digestive problems, and the like, without considering that these ailments are often symptoms of depression. They keep patients on an "average" dosage, but dosage requirements are highly variable from person to person. Many doctors don't suggest switching to another antidepressant if the one first prescribed doesn't do the trick within six weeks, or, alternatively, they discontinue a medication before it has a chance to work. The track record of psychiatrists is better, but even they often fail to distinguish between typical and atypical depression (about which you will learn more later in this chapter), thus condemning as high as 40 percent of all depressed patients to a semi-encouraging six months, followed by a descent once again into the pits. The top performers are the psychopharmacologists, who specialize in the medical treatment of psychiatric illness and keep abreast of the latest research on drugs and treatment. Among them are some world-class depression detectives whose skill and expertise justify their fees. The very best among them are the first to admit that treating depression is still as much an art as a science.

## The Unofficial Symptoms List

The doctor's checklist of symptoms is of some help to fall-out partners, but it can easily lead them to the faulty conclusion that a partner's depression does indeed stem from a troubled relationship, and their own role in it, rather than the other way around. After all, everyone has occasional trouble with sleeping and appetite; everyone gets irritable from time to time; everyone, including men, will occasionally cry; and hardly anyone is interested in sex all the time. Today's racing pace is enough to stun a horse, so fatigue seems the norm, and it's hard to find a person who doesn't suffer from headaches or lower back pain. I have long since concluded that most depression professionals never cohabit with depressed people or, if they do, fail to recognize that their partners' at-home behavior doesn't concur with the cool and objective list of symptoms by which they judge their patients.

My claim to symptom expertise comes from being both a depression fallout sufferer and a triple-A depressive myself, and is amplified and illuminated by a greedy appetite for listening to the experiences of others on each side of the fence. Before reading the list of unofficial symptoms, rid yourself of that stereotypic image of a depressed person as someone who sits quietly on the sidelines look-ing sad and forlorn. "Sad" is a misleading description of how this illness feels; "deadened by apathy," "floating in a gray, emotionless void," and "laboring under the secret conviction that life offers neither hope nor rewards" come closer to the mark. Depression fallout observers, unable to access their partners' despairing inner thoughts, may judge their behavior less dispassionately and recognize the following as an accurate description of their mates:

- self-absorbed, selfish, demanding, unaware or uncon-cerned about the needs of others

- unresponsive, uncommunicative, aloof, withdrawn

- uninterested in sex and dismissive or distrusting of a partner's tenderness and affection

- fractious, querulous, combative, contrary; finding fault with everything

- demeaning and critical of partner

- changeable and unpredictable; illogical and unreason-able

- manipulative

- pleasant and charming in public and the opposite at home

- prone to sudden, inexplicable references to separation or divorce

- prone to workaholism or avoidance of all responsibility

- increasingly dependent on alcohol and drugs

- obsessively addicted to television, computer games and computer porn sites, and other compulsive distractions

Although all depressions share common characteristics, they come individually fingerprinted by the genes, temperament, and environment of each sufferer. One depression sufferer may call in sick and then while away the daytime hours by gobbling ordered-in pizza and dozing in front of the television, then, still in his bathrobe, wander around the house all night. Another leaves for her office at seven in the morning and comes home late, using an overwhelming workload to explain why there is no dinner for the family and no chitchat for her mate. Neither is sociable in the sense of seeking human contact for enjoyment's sake, but both are capable of acting "normally" in public and then swiftly reverting to an aloof hostility once inside the front door. This dichotomy between public and private personae tops the fallout list of most resented behaviors. What could be more hurtful than a partner who gratuitously displays affection at a party and then stiffens and withdraws from advances later that night in bed?

Approximately half of all first episodes of depression spontaneously remit in six to nine months, never to return. If the first episode is followed by a second, the likelihood of a third episode rises to about 80 percent; with each return visit, the depression becomes more severe and also more resistant to treatment. Some depressions are chronic and some are treatment resistant, but this illness more commonly waxes and wanes; some days, or even weeks, may be marked by a somewhat improved mood, which then dissipates.

Most of its sufferers (including me) have a repertoire of seemingly conflicting behaviors—very difficult for us to control—that alternately raise and dash the hopes of partners, who portray themselves as tiptoeing on eggshells to avoid yet another confrontation or as being trapped on an out-of-control roller coaster. From their fallout vantage point, these unofficial symptoms resemble the acquisition of new bad habits and the abandonment of good old ones, all at a whim. The notion that they are caused by an illness seems outlandish, especially since, with the exception of noticeable changes in sleeping and eating patterns and in energy levels, they are unaccompanied by the clues provided by most physical ailments. But the sadly immutable fact is that depression has the power to profoundly alter attitudes and behavior. Suggesting to its victims that they have much to be thankful for and should pull up their socks is counterproductive. They would do so if they could.

## DEPRESSION'S CLOSE RELATIVES

Depression is often mistakenly used as a blanket term for a number of less common psychiatric illnesses that belong to the same family. Prime among them is *manic depression,* which afflicts about 2.3 million people in the United States and is the most dangerous, disabling, and hardest to treat. This cruel illness is also called *bipolar disorder* because its sufferers alternate between depressed lows and manic highs (unipolar depressives visit only the downs). Some bipolars spend months or even years in the depths of despair before soaring unexpectedly into the heights of mania; others take the reverse route, first rising, then sinking, or periodically alternating between the two extremes.

When in a manic phase, bipolars are blissfully unaware of how bizarre their behavior appears to onlookers. They feel on top of the world, suffused with feelings of invincibility, well-being, and limitless energy, but these come packaged with aggressiveness, extreme irritability, and bursts of anger that may translate into violence. When the fall comes, manic depressives are sincerely appalled by the damage they have caused, but, like cocaine addicts, they retain siren memories of the grandeur and glory that once were theirs. Even when the crash is preceded by delusional psychosis and followed by hospitalization, they often willingly forsake the medications prescribed—many of which have extremely unpleasant side effects—and the devastating cycle begins all over again.

The official symptoms of mania, which need be present for only one week to receive the diagnosis, are as follows:

- inappropriate elation or irritability

- decreased need for sleep

- increased energy

- increased talking, moving, and sexual activity

- racing thoughts

- grandiose notions

- disturbed ability to make decisions

A complete list of mania's unofficial symptoms embraces extremist and delusional behaviors. During its onset in your partner, your initial reaction may be a matching sense of exhilaration, and your interpretation might be that your mate has found a new enthusiasm for living. If, for example, she is normally reticent, you will delight in her desire to chat nonstop, until you realize she talks right over your replies. If he has been hard to roust out of bed each morning, you will be pleased to see him up and running at five, until you note that it's twenty hours later and he is still at top speed. But when they buy thirty identical pairs of sneakers, wipe out your joint bank account to buy a discredited stock, decide to run for Congress or write the great American novel, and start sleeping around but not with you, the impact will be emotionally and financially devastating.

Untreated, over-the-top mania spins into psychosis and usually ends in the emergency room. The mother of a high-strung, budding concert pianist noted at breakfast one morning that her daughter seemed extremely agitated and promised to leave the office early to look after her. On return she found an empty apartment in alarming disarray. Hours later, with the help of the police, her daughter was discovered wandering the wintry streets in a T-shirt, talking to herself and terrified of everyone, including her mother, who tried to coax her into an ambulance. This manic episode was cut short by early intervention; often discovery comes only after far greater damage has been done.

Manic depression has subsets, among them *cyclothymia*, a less extreme, chronic form of manic depression. While cyclothymia also requires a lifelong regimen of drugs, its sufferers are spared the extremes, gyrating instead between mildish highs and lows that cannot be predicted with any certainty. *Hypomania* is the only relatively benign member of the manic-depressive family. Thoroughly enjoyable to have around, and presenting few problems for spouses and partners (unless they are hermits or Zen Buddhists), hypomanics are often high achievers and good leaders, imaginative and productive, and possess a winning charm and unlimited self-confidence. If that sounds like the description of a skilled bond trader, a supersalesperson, or a winning politician, it is because hypomanics are attracted to careers that make good use of their disorder.

*Dysthymia* is the disagreeable opposite of hypomania, a low-grade, chronic version of depression, perhaps even more disheartening than the real thing because it is unremitting. Many dysthymics never seek or receive an accurate diagnosis because, rather than appearing "mentally ill," they resemble people we try to avoid because they are so relentlessly negative and humorless. Instead of indulging in classic depressive behavior—which might alert someone to their plight—they sip away from their

half-empty glass until, sometimes years later, they drink it
dry and plummet downward into full-fledged depression.
Dysthymia's symptoms (only two or more, providing they
have been present for at least two years), which will
ensure a diagnosis by an expert, but not necessarily by a
less experienced practitioner, are as follows:

- poor appetite or overeating

- insomnia or hypersomnia

- low energy or fatigue

- low self-esteem

- poor concentration or difficulty making decisions

- feelings of hopelessness

*Atypical depression,* my own affliction, is a grievously
underdiagnosed sibling of depression with its own set of
symptoms. Some of the differences between depression
and atypical depression are physical: atypical sufferers
sleep excessively, overeat, and gain weight due to our
neurotransmitter-driven desire for high-carbohydrate foods
such as butter-laden bread and pasta, candy, rich desserts,
and French fries. We also have two psychological anomalies:
If dragged to a party, we actually enjoy ourselves, only to
deflate like pricked balloons on returning home; we retain
no memory of these good times and, so, experience no pleasurable anticipation of future ones. The second is an overwhelming sensitivity to rejection that, although unrelated to
reality, shapes all our interpersonal relations. Constantly

bombarded by imagined major and minor slights, we seek evidence that we are worthy of attention, praise, approval, and love, but when others do love and admire us, we doubt their motives and are unwilling to believe them.

Last in this abridged primer of mood disorders are the *anxiety disorders,* which are clustered around specific types of behavior; they are often harbingers and then partners of depression. *Panic disorder* is characterized by sudden, irrational feelings of fear and dread that make the heart pound wildly; in the midst of an acute panic attack it's hard to breathe and easy to think "I'm going to die." An example of the presence of generalized panic disorder is provided by a busy, overbooked person who takes a forty-mile, back-road detour twice a day to avoid fifteen minutes on the freeway. Unless panic disorder is diagnosed and treated, it may result in agoraphobia, which ultimately can render its sufferers so terrified of leaving home base that they become isolated and reclusive.

*Obsessive-compulsive disorder* forces its sufferers to wash their hands until they are raw, to check over and over again that the gas really is turned off and the front door locked, and to churn every thought as though the mind was trapped on an unstoppable treadmill. Jack Nicholson's character in the film *As Good As It Gets,* who had to arrange knife, fork, spoon, salt, glass, and napkin in exactly the same pattern before eating the same meal every day, served by the same waitress at the same table in the same coffee shop, exemplifies this disorder.

*Generalized anxiety disorder* is a serious illness and usually precedes or accompanies depression. Run-of-the-mill anxiety is a normal fact of life, but the disorder of that name far surpasses job jitters and worries that your child's poor grades will keep him or her out of Yale. In addition to physical symptoms such as muscle tension and incessant worrying, the clinically anxious are not reassured by a promotion at work, a child's straight A's, or a good mammogram report. Women are more predisposed to anxiety than men (no one knows why); once afflicted, both sexes almost invariably move on to depression and may end up with a newly classified disorder known as *mixed anxiety-depression.*

## NOTES FROM THE UNDERGROUND: WHAT YOUR DEPRESSED PERSON IS REALLY THINKING

Fallout partners need to constantly remind themselves that the behavior they witness is driven by an illness. Subtle changes in the functioning of brain chemicals do indeed explain why your depressed partner retreats from your embrace, is thoughtless and critical, and snaps for no reason at you and the kids. Acceptance of this indisputable fact is the best fallout shield against self-blame, demoralization, and resentment. Depression is a no-fault illness; no one purposely invites or enjoys being depressed, and blaming your partner for having inherited a genetic vulnerability is preposterous and unrewarding. Why so many depressed people deny their illness and refuse professional help is addressed in the next chapter; in the meantime, a privileged look at their fiercely guarded interior landscape may surprise you and also help you communicate better with them.

Michele posted her "Underground" list of symptoms on the Message Board under the heading "What depression means to me":

- Depression means disappointing people by not living up to their expectations of me.

- It means waking up each morning and dreading the day.

- It means failure—failure in everything I do.

- It means living like a hermit—shutting my phone off, shutting the world out.

- It means living with such guilt—feeling guilty of things that are out of my control.

- It means sleeping too much—I sleep so I can escape.

- It means feeling like the whole world is closing in on me.

- It means ALWAYS having negative thoughts.

- It means however much you pray, God doesn't answer your prayers.

- It means letting relationships go.

- It means thinking that at any moment something bad will happen again.

Like Michele, many, perhaps most, depression sufferers are ashamed of the feelings that motivate these symptoms and erect what she refers to as "The Wall" to hide them from intimates. The safety zone thus created is usually defended by silence, but sometimes even a casual "How do you feel?" can unleash a startling reply. A recently divorced Board poster received an E-mail response from her depressed ex-husband that was totally at odds with the obstreperous, selfish behavior that had finally led to their divorce. "May you never find out what it's like to not know or recognize or understand yourself or your motivations, and worst of all, to hate what you see in yourself," he wrote. "I turned into a horrible person, and although I know that, I can't stop it or change it," which, he added, was why it had been easier for him to leave her than to stay married. "Am I happier now? No, but at least I can be miserable without ruining someone else's life."

Such damning self-judgments are rarely voiced to partners, even when the family is in turmoil and the prospect of separation or divorce is imminent. A few of the scrappy notes I penned while floating in my own gray void hint at a similar existential angst, but retroactive portrayals of "how it felt" are seldom reliable. The selective action of memory, combined with effective medication, act as broom and soap to pretty up the detritus of a once severely depressed psyche. Far more revealing are unedited communications straight from the battlefront, as anyone who has visited a depression chat room knows.

The Message Board is blessed with occasional depression war correspondents. One of them, Paul, a divorced, depressed father of two, over the course of a month courageously put his psyche on display and answered some fallout queries usually met by argumentative non sequiturs:

"Why are you so illogical and contradictory?" "Why do you keep telling me to leave you alone?" "Why do you get so angry at me when all I want to do is help you?" "Why do you behave as though you don't love me anymore?" Stroke by stroke, Paul created a generic portrait of a mind locked in depression. "The way we think and behave is part of the illness, and the illness doesn't reason," he explained. "When it's in charge, everything we say and do makes perfect sense to us, so we're puzzled when others don't understand us. We do the things we do in the same way that a heart beats, effortlessly, without conscious instructions, so we don't notice anything is wrong. When we act 'strangely,' it isn't about what you may or may not have said or done; it's about a brain that is not working right."

Paul went on to acknowledge that being in a committed relationship requires that each partner be emotionally "there" for the other, but that the effort is more than the depressed can handle. "My preferred companion is my cat because he sits patiently across the room, waiting until I feel like spending time with him, and when I'm done, I walk away and that's fine with Cat. From our skewed viewpoint, if you don't want to be with us when we need you, you are being selfish, and if you need us when we aren't ready to give, you are being demanding. When the darkness lifts, we don't understand why you're unhappy with us." But often with the lifting comes the realization of having hurt an innocent person, bringing guilt and contrition that are hard to face and even harder to express. "I know then that I don't deserve love, and that my depression is screwing up not just my own life, but my wife's and my daughters' as well. I find no words, no way to tell them that, or to convey my guilt."

I was never a diarist, though I did jot down notes about the way I felt in particularly sad or happy moments. I was also a prodigious collector of letters written and received from various lovers, all of which I stashed in a box marked "Old Ramblings." Suspecting the contents might yield an explanatory footnote to Paul's guilt, I dug it out from the back of the closet and came upon an age-yellowed carbon copy of a letter to my then adored boyfriend apologizing for my compulsively angry behavior. "When things go wrong between us," I explained, "they arise from my actions and my problems, not from yours. I feel so very guilty for hurting you. I do love you, but every time I see you the guilt and self-hatred come on strong, which in turn makes me even angrier with myself and more guilty, and this goes on and on in a vicious circle." Paul, in trying to explain the reasonless anger of depression, explained that quite a lot of it is really directed inward, "but we need to release it somehow. We direct it at those we love because, whether consciously or unconsciously, we know they love us back and will go on forgiving us for a long time."

If asked to rank depression's symptoms on a scale of 1 to 10, uncontrollable anger would score an 11. In my Ramblings box is a scrawled note, penned on returning from a since-forgotten evening. I have no idea what ignited my anger, but I wrote that it was "rip-roaring, out of control," leaving me breathless, outraged, and murderous. "Vicious winds fill me. I mustn't allow anyone to see me like this," I cautioned myself, and then, several hours later, noted that the "cyclone" was gone, leaving me weak but calmer. "It's moved from my stomach to my mind. When it went, it left a void and now I have no feelings at all. I am no longer 'the same person.' How do I feel? Back on square one, no progress."

I would never describe myself as placid and unemotional, but the pent up, irrational rage with which I lived frightened me back then, as it must frighten many depression sufferers; it had a life and a will of its own and usually took me by surprise. Although cyclones were reserved for grand occasions, even passing encounters with strangers—a supermarket clerk or a check-in agent at the airport—could raise my temperature and set me to muttering, "Shit, shit, shit." I knew I was acting like a deranged person, but like so much of depressed behavior, I couldn't stop it. Accusations of our illogicality and irrationality are fully justified; and so, in a sense, is our claim that they are not our fault. In a poem written for the Message Board entitled "Nothing at All," Paul conveys our sense that we are puppets manipulated by an invisible, malign master.

> Sometimes I sit and wonder
> What happened to my life's direction
> My happiness and vigor
> Lost to depression
> I can't go back and make it better
> I hope yet cannot change the way you feel
> Said and done you're still the one
> But I'm trapped on this wheel

I thought you would see
I thought you would know
I didn't lose the love
Only how to show it

A number of books by depression sufferers attempt to convey how it feels to be depressed. One of the earliest written is William Styron's *Darkness Visible: A Memoir of Madness,* mentioned earlier. His illness, which he acknowledges had doubtless been hovering for years, swooped down during a faultless summer on Martha's Vineyard. As it settled, he began to "respond indifferently to the island's pleasures." "I felt a kind of numbness," he writes, "an enervation, but more particularly an odd fragility—as if my body had actually become frail, hypersensitive, and somehow disjointed and clumsy. . . . Nothing felt quite right with my corporeal self; there were twitches and pains, sometimes intermittent, often seemingly constant, that seemed to presage all sorts of dire infirmities." Casting light on the symptom of aches and pains for which doctors find no cause, Styron sees them as "part of the psyche's apparatus of defense: unwilling to accept its own gathering deterioration, the mind announces to its indwelling consciousness that it is the body with its perhaps correctable defects—not the precious and irreplaceable mind—that is going haywire." He was particularly aware of the "lamentable near disappearance" of his voice, which underwent a transformation, "becoming at times quite faint, wheezy and spasmodic," and was later characterized by a friend as that of a ninety-year-old. An anonymous writer once described this state as feeling as though she was wrapped in cotton wool, and that she heard her own voice echoing strangely, as though coming from outer space.

Vivid thoughts of suicide—of how and when to do it—surface in despairing minds. William Styron likens this to "the sense of being accompanied by a second self—a wraithlike observer who, not sharing the dementia of his double, is able to watch with dispassionate curiosity as his companion struggles against the oncoming disaster, or decides to embrace it." He set about rewriting his will and tried to compose a suitable suicide note, but could manage neither the "dirgelike solemnity," nor the numerous "final bouquets" he felt obliged to offer to his wife and to his many friends. Later, as he sat miserably in the living room watching a taped movie with a classical music sound track, a passage from Brahms's *Alto Rhapsody* "pierced my heart like a dagger, and in a flood of swift recollection I thought of all the joys the house had known." He woke up his wife and the next day was admitted to the hospital, a hopeful ending to a story of serious depression.

Kay Redfield Jamison, a professor of psychiatry at Johns Hopkins University and a leading authority on bipolar illness, knows her subject both professionally and personally. In *An Unquiet Mind: A Memoir of Moods and Madness,* she describes her first personal encounter with manic depression when a senior in high school, quite unlike what she calls the "true" mania of her college and later years. "At first, everything seemed so easy," she writes. "I raced about like a crazed weasel, bubbling with plans and enthusiasms, immersed in sports, and staying up all night, night after night, out with friends, reading everything that wasn't nailed down, filling manuscript books with poems and fragments of plays, and making expansive, completely unrealistic, plans for my future. The world was filled with pleasure and promise; I felt great." Jamison cautions that feeling great is no more an accurate description of mania than is feeling sad for depression. In mania, Kay Jamison felt *really* great, so great that she felt she could accomplish anything, that no task was beyond for her. "My mind seemed clear, fabulously focused, and able to make intuitive mathematical leaps that had up to that point entirely eluded me. . . . [N]ot only did everything make perfect sense, but it all began to fit into a marvelous kind of cosmic relatedness. My sense of enchantment with the laws of the natural world caused me to fizz over, and I found myself buttonholing my friends to tell them how beautiful it all was."

Her friends, less "transfixed" than Kay by her insights into "the webbings and beauties of the universe," told her to slow down. Their warnings didn't make a dent, but then her mood turned upside down and depression took over. First came boredom and a complete indifference to life, soon followed by a "gray, bleak preoccupation with death, dying, decaying, [and the thought] that everything was born but to die, best to die now and save the pain while waiting. . . . I aged rapidly during those months, as one must with such loss of one's self, with such proximity to death, and such distance from shelter."

These and other similar books have attracted millions of readers, many of whom surely recognize themselves within the covers. Yet I would wager a year's supply of my save-me-from-this-fate antidepressants that only a handful rushed to the phone to call a doctor. The efficiency of the depressed and manic mind in blocking out the most strident clues, why this is so, and what you can do about it are the subjects of the next chapter.

# 3

# Overcoming Denial: The Art of Persuasion

The swiftest route to ending depression fallout before entering stage five is to persuade your partner that he or she suffers from depression and needs professional help. If on your first attempt you were able to pull off this feat—described by a Board poster as the Oscar-Winning Dream of the Year—stop reading and write a post that explains in mind-boggling detail how you chose your moment; how you approached the subject; what you received in the way of a response; what arguments you used to overcome disclaimers, objections, and opinions to the contrary; and how you celebrated your remarkable victory. If, on the other hand, mere mention of the word *depression* ignited an uncelebratory bonfire, welcome to another meeting of the Seriously Confused Club. The term of your membership in the club will depend on the severity and duration of the illness; your skill, tact, and patience; and the degree of your familiarity with the illogical thinking processes of the depressed—plus a dollop of luck.

According to the law of averages, there must be depressed men and women out there who listen quietly to their partners' words, then say, "You know, you're right, I haven't been feeling like myself lately and I'll call the doctor right now," and even a few who express their gratitude to a clever, loving mate for having put a finger on the source of some recent problems between them. A more likely response is outraged denial followed by an attack on your sanity. Some winning strategies for overcoming denial follow an explanation of what causes it.

## THE POWER OF STIGMAS AND STEREOTYPES

Assertions of denial will be repeated over weeks, months, or even longer unless you apply yourself to the art of persuasion. The reasons for this extend beyond sheer pigheadedness. Denial of depression is rooted in long-held societal stereotypes that persist despite torrents of information proving them incorrect and outdated. Type "depression" into a computer search engine and up pops a year's worth of 24/7 reading. Type "denial of depression" into www.google.com and choose among the 94,100 possibilities offered. Why, then, do the vast majority of its victims, and often their families as well, continue to view this illness as shameful? When Happy Rockefeller, the wife of then-governor of New York State Nelson Rockefeller, publicly revealed that she had breast cancer, millions of women stopped being secretive about their fear and began having annual mammograms. When Betty Ford revealed that she had a drinking problem, alcoholism came to be seen as a treatable illness rather than self-indulgence. Elizabeth Taylor and Governor Dukakis's wife, Kitty, changed the image of drug addiction when they admitted to a dependency on painkillers. But when accurate rumors of Princess Diana's depression began to circulate, they were adamantly denied by the Royal Family and steadfastly ignored by her devoted public. Remarkably enough, the rules of today's cockeyed world seem to be: If you are a famous substance abuser, admit it; if you suffer from depression, bury it.

Fallout partners who are baffled by adamant denial will find a partial explanation in the experiences of some headliners who, rightfully as it turned out, feared disclosure of their illness. Tipper Gore, an early warrior in the fight to destigmatize mental illness and put it on a par with physical illness, demonstrated great courage when, during her husband's campaign for the presidency, she acknowledged having turned to antidepressants and psychotherapy to cope with their son's near-fatal car accident. Although she also freely acknowledged her mother's long battle with apathy and hopelessness, Mrs. Gore sidestepped the questions that followed; her reticence was soon justified. Investigative reporters dug up the document her father had filed in seeking a divorce from Tipper's mother; among its claims was the assertion that his wife was of a "nervous, volatile, flighty and erratic temperament" and "so lacking in normal maternal instincts" that she was sometimes unable to get out of bed in the morning to take care of their fourteen-month-old baby, Tipper. A subsequent *New*

*York Times* feature article stopped short of stating that Mrs. Gore still relies on medication and instead dropped clues about her mood swings, implying instability.

Wild conspiracy theories still cloak the suicide of Clinton Presidential aide Vince Foster, who killed himself because his serious depression blotted out all other options. During Michael Dukakis's run for the presidency, an unfounded rumor that he had consulted a psychiatrist after his brother's death drove his polls down eight points in two days. *New York Times* columnist Frank Rich, an ardent anti-stigma advocate, reported Ronald Reagan's below-the-belt comment at the time—that he wasn't going to "pick on an invalid"; the elder George Bush's campaign manager chimed in, saying "real men don't get on the couch." An earlier horror story was the discarding of Senator Thomas Eagleton from the 1972 Democratic ticket after his revelation of once having been hospitalized for depression, which caused former secretary of the interior Bruce Babbitt to warn politicians many years later: "Don't go near a psychiatrist. It's the kiss of death."

The policy powerhouses behind the Mental Health Parity Act (at present, mental illnesses receive a fraction of the reimbursements offered for physical illnesses), Senators Paul Wellstone and Pete Domenici, who both have a close relative with mental illness, have been unable for five years to pass the bill because of conservative resistance. One glimmer of hope is the winning campaign of Congresswoman Lynn Rivers, who first spoke publicly about her long battle with manic depression in the closing days of her campaign—and won a second term. When a caller, possibly planted by her opponent, asked her on a radio talk show if she'd ever "had a problem" with depression, she answered, "Absolutely! Millions and millions of people do."

Being an author is perhaps the sole career in which success is guaranteed by telling the world that one has this illness, providing the writer in question is super-famous and widely admired. Sports provide a harsh contrast; the few players who have admitted to depression find the free agent waters chilly or frozen over. The entertainment world is less concerned about the moods of its stars, but even so, actress Margot Kidder's public breakdown invited headlines and voyeurism that a diagnosis of cancer or a heart attack would never have provoked. In industry and financial circles, psychiatric illness of any kind is verboten. Rude, raw, and often outrageous, business genius Ted Turner has been making news and mountains of money for twenty years without a public statement from him concerning the manic depression he inherited from his father; shareholders would see it as evidence of instability and unreliability.

File clerks worry about being fired for unreliability and parents about being declared unfit, just as Kay Redfield Jamison worried that publication of her memoir might cause her professional peers to discount her work. Face up to the probability that your partner is similarly worried, and that overcoming his or her denial will be a long haul. Your understanding of how the brain directs the mind's emotional and cognitive traffic will tip the odds of success in your favor.

## WHAT DOES DENIAL LOOK LIKE
## UP CLOSE AND PERSONAL?

It is not humanly possible to be depressed without knowing that something is wrong; disagreement over who or
what is responsible is where your challenge will start. For
a variety of reasons, never begin your conversation by saying, "I think you're depressed." No doubt when the term
"depression" was first adopted it seemed a giant step up
from "mentally disturbed" because it correctly differenti-
ates between illness and madness. Yet to many, this term
still has connotations of loony bins and wild-haired cra-
zies. Today's politically correct world puts the emphasis
on mental health rather than mental illness; unfortunately, suggesting that your mate is mentally unhealthy
will sound more like an accusation of sexual deviance than
of being depressed, but there are alternative openers.

### The Oscar-Winning Scenario

The safest opening to your campaign might be something
along the lines of "I've been noticing lately that you're not
sleeping well at night. Are they working you too hard at
the office?" or "You're usually such a pussycat, but
recently you've been edgy and kind of irritable," followed
again by the office problem line, or, if there isn't an office
to blame, substitute boisterous children, difficult in-laws
(preferably your parents), the state of the stock market, or
the pressing need for roof repairs or a new car. The rationale for calling attention to sleep disturbances is that they

coexist with depression but are not threatening to the ego. If the words *edgy* and *irritable* are preceded by a compliment, they are less likely to set off fireworks than if voiced as a complaint on your part.

As always when tackling a problem with someone who is depressed, choose your moment carefully. Never bring up the topic when your spouse is angry, or when you are in the middle of an argument, or when the children or other people are present. If much of the time you spend together now borders on the tense, wait for a neutral moment, perhaps after you have been to a good movie together and the atmosphere is relatively untroubled. Do not try to capitalize on extraneous good news—your partner's losing football team has won a game or her business deal is progressing well; the depressed react badly if you rain on their parade. Pay attention to your body language; rather than crossing your arms tightly over your chest, adopt your normal everything-is-okay posture and look pleasantly at your partner, not at your feet. Keep your tone of voice chatty and affectionate.

In a perfect world, the one where your dream wins the Oscar, your partner will admit to sleeping poorly lately (or needing more of it than usual), to loss of appetite, and to feeling pressured and stressed out at times. Encourage him or her to come up with the "reasons" for this, be they office, kids, money problems, or whatever is germane, and keep the conversation going until they have talked themselves out. This is your opportunity to nudge closer to depression by saying, "Do you remember that article a couple of months ago in *Newsweek* (you are on firm ground here as every publication and media outlet regularly runs stories on the topic) about depression and how many people have it? I didn't pay much attention at the time, but I do remember that sleeping and eating problems and feeling edgy are signs of it." Your spouse or lover may reply that people who can't solve their problems are deadbeats, a statement you can counter by citing Woody Allen, Judy Garland, J. P. Morgan, Eleanor Roosevelt, Patricia Cornwell, and Winston Churchill, a few on the long list of depressed high achievers in every walk of life. Having planted the seed, drop the subject for a few days, then reintroduce it after the next sleepless night or a weekend spent conked out on the sofa. As before, focus on depression's physical symptoms and emphasize your concern about their potential to curb your mate's enjoyment and concentration. Gradually add more information about depression and admit you have been reading up on it because you care about your partner. By sticking to your guns and keeping your approach low-key and nonconfrontational, you may succeed.

You know your partner better than anyone else. Tailor your precise strategy to suit his or her character and the relationship style that has evolved over time. Nagging and harping, accusations of foot-dragging, and a resentful attitude will not serve you well. Avoid questions such as "Do you still love me?" "Why are you acting so cold?" and "What's the matter with you, is it us?" as they will derail the discussion and send it into dangerous byways. A cautionary word about sex (covered more fully in Chapter 7) is in order here. Depression inhibits the libido, inducing tension and unhappiness on the part of both partners. Even if sex is still rewarding, a post-intercourse discussion about depression, no matter how it's introduced, is risky as it may raise the specter of impotency lurking in your partner's mind, as yet unshared with you. If occasionally you are offered gestures of affection, enjoy them as proof that you are still loved despite your fears. Your goal is to get your partner to make an appointment with a doctor, not with a marriage counselor.

These scripted scenarios, and their stage directions in regard to body language and tone of voice, should be followed even when depressed partners make theirs up on the spot. The prototypical response lines are provocative and guaranteed to raise your temper. Keep it at any price.

## FAVORITE UNSCRIPTED DENIAL LINES

The Message Board is rife with posts concerning denial dialogues, referred to as "Conversations with the Sphinx" and "News from the Twilight Zone." Board posters put together a list of some typical comebacks uttered by their depressed mates:

- I don't know what you're talking about.

- I haven't time to talk about this now.

- Don't worry, I can handle it.

- All I need is some time to myself.

- So I'm having trouble sleeping/am tired, what's the big deal?

- I had a physical last month and the doctor said I was just fine.

- Thanks for making my day.

- You'd rather drug me into being someone I'm not than admit that you might have some issues.

- If anyone's depressed around here it's you.

- The real problem is us, not me.

All of the above represent a facade behind which lie fear, a drooping self-esteem, and guilt for behaving badly. Your depressed person knows something is wrong but is reluctant to find out what that might be. Unlike physical illnesses that demand immediate attention and medical help, depression has symptoms that are easily explained away; your partner will avoid thinking about them until they are so disabling that they stand up and shout for attention. In depression's moderate forms, a streak of bad days will be preceded and followed by a few good ones. These cyclical rhythms lull sufferers into believing that it was a false alarm and now all is well again forever.

As for last month's physical, it probably included blood, urine, and other standard tests, a lung X ray, and an EKG to check out the heart. For the unexplained aches, pains, and stomach distress that often accompany depression, most physicians order tests only to find nothing wrong. Complaints of being fatigued or overly anxious are often rewarded with prescriptions for sleeping pills and antianxiety drugs. In short, unless the physician is experienced, the standard HMO physical does not reveal depression unless the patient volunteers information relevant to its diagnosis.

The psychological symptoms—feelings of hopelessness, helplessness, and toying, no matter how briefly, with the idea of suicide—are zealously guarded secrets. The depression sufferer tackles low self-esteem by repeated vows to get it together, be nicer, start working out more, make better use of time, and thus beat the rat race conveniently blamed for the malaise. The most powerful silencer is fear of projecting the image of someone incapable of solving problems on his or her own: an unmanly weakling, a woman unable to handle both her family and her work, crybabies not strong enough to make it in a competitive world. To be labeled thus due to a mental illness for which one must take medicine is alarming. Add feelings of guilt and unworthiness, and the mix becomes toxic. Although it may not look that way, your depressed partner is upset and worried that you may bail out and leave him or her stranded in the gray fog.

What strengthens many people's denial is a deep suspicion of drugs that can "control the mind." One depressed reader asked for advice on how to treat her depression other than with medication because she didn't believe that changing neurochemistry was a good thing unless done "naturally." Heavy drinkers and smokers suddenly adopt a pious my-body-is-a-temple attitude when told to take a daily pill. Surely willpower is safer than medications that meddle with the brain, runs their argument, and surely resorting to drugs to control one's feelings is the ultimate in weakness.

## WINNING STRATEGIES

The essential prerequisite for winning is a cool head and an even temper. Comments like "Thanks for making my day" and "Don't worry, I can handle it" are designed to shift the focus off depression and onto your putative failings as a partner. Denying that you are the one who is depressed and the troublemaker invites anecdotes, retold in excruciating detail, about the time last February when you forgot to pick up milk on the way home, or slept through church, or wouldn't make love, or any of the petty resentments your mate has been storing up. Defending yourself by listing your partner's misdeeds will serve his or her purpose well, even though it means an argument at the kindergarten level.

Staying on track requires one of the following responses: "Considering how many people *are* depressed, maybe we're in the same boat. Maybe we should both check it out with a doctor"; "Your complaints may be valid, but right now I'm telling you that I'm worried about your lack of sleep"; or "Of course I don't think you're crazy, but I do think you're getting less fun out of life lately." All will bring the temperature down and make way for another bullet of information: the ten billion spent annually on antidepressants in the United States, the best-selling books on depression, the famous high achievers like Richard Rodgers, F. Scott Fitzgerald, Audrey Hepburn, and Virginia Woolf. Be ready to back off the "depression is prevalent" approach if it provokes hostility; some depression sufferers may think their individuality is being questioned. Instead, say something like "I am used to you being a very motivated person, but lately you've been leaving some basic things undone."

The killer denial is "The real problem is us, not me" and it stars in many Message Board dramas. A husband posting under the name Forever opens by asking how he can get his wife to acknowledge that her frequent office crying jags and sleepless nights are due to depression, "that it is more than 'us.'" Married for eight years and with a two-year-old, they had always considered themselves the happiest couple in their circle, but now, despite six months of persuasion on Forever's part, his wife insists her tears and loss of sleep and appetite are signs of a marital problem, and that the only solution is divorce. "She says that everything else in her life is okay, so how could she possibly be clinically depressed?" he writes. "Her sudden emotional shift and willingness to give up the life we have built and the future we have planned, plus all of the symptoms she has shown, truly make me believe she is suffering from some kind of clinical depression."

While Forever is right, his repetitive use of the word *clinical*, probably also used in conversation with his wife, may have sounded threatening to her and been one reason that his campaign has been unsuccessful thus far. Her physical symptoms, without making any reference to depression, merited a visit to the doctor if for no other reason than to ask for a mild sedative. Although his wife did see a physician, and even allowed her husband to accompany her, she adamantly refused to take an antidepressant if prescribed because, she insisted, she had no problem other than unhappiness with him. Forever presented his "case" to the doctor: his wife's abrupt change of heart, her uncontrollable weeping, loss of appetite and of weight, the nights spent tossing and turning, and other clear signs of depression. Her "case" was to stubbornly repeat that she was happy in all aspects of life outside their relationship. The physician displayed his ignorance of depression's symptoms and causes by recommending marriage counseling instead of antidepressants. If Forever had been privy to the advice offered above and done the necessary groundwork, a more appropriate diagnosis might have been made, one that did not reinforce his wife's belief that their marriage had gone bad.

Bizarre as this story may sound, even more irrational versions of the us-versus-me denial are a staple of depression fallout. "I've heard that 'I'm just not happy with our relationship' jazz a zillion times," writes Katie. "One day my depressed husband sent me a one-line E-mail saying, 'I am very bitter and I quit,' nothing else. What did he suppose I was going to gather from that statement? Quit what? His life? His job? His marriage? If it's marriage, that would be a new tack, but then again, I gather from you folks on the Board that it shouldn't be a big surprise." Katie's turndown of a lunch invitation to discuss "their" problem was a wise decision, not only because her husband had been simmering with bitterness for days and refused to talk civilly at home but also because she knew she was too angry to keep on her kid gloves. "I refuse to engage in war mode," she continues. "I must manage my own anger before I allow him to create even more fallout."

One hopes, however, that after temporarily exorcising her anger by pounding the pillows or taking a run, Katie took advantage of her husband's next offer to talk. By pre-scripting her part of the dialogue, progress might be made.

The eeriest example of this mindset is a post by Margaret, whose husband of twelve years declared that they should sep-arate just as she was being wheeled into the delivery room to give birth to their third child. His pronouncement did not come without warning; several months earlier her husband had declared that his "inner essence" told him it was time to exit their marriage. Remarkably, other posters admitted to similar crises that coincided with pregnancy events—testimony to the depression sufferer's depleted capacity to handle major life changes. Efforts to hold the family together for the children's sake and to restore a loving relationship may sometimes succeed, but patience and fortitude can be taken to extremes. Margaret says she looks for little victories along the way, but critical signs of instability should be chal-lenged immediately. Margaret missed what could have been the greatest victory of all: persuading her husband that, given the magnitude of his doubts and their implications for the family, it was imperative that he submit his decision to the judgment of an "impartial" psychologist or family counselor.

## Getting Inside Your Partner's Head

Denial is the strongest of all defense mechanisms, and although it has a negative reputation, in some instances it serves a useful purpose. One example is when a bereaved spouse refuses for months to accept that the partner is truly gone and then, as he or she grows psychologically stronger, accepts the loss and begins rebuilding a life. Fallout sufferers practice benign denial when they repeat over and over again, "This is no longer the person I fell in love with." But the brand of denial adopted by depressives is closer to the denial practiced by alcohol and drug abusers, who refuse to accept the addiction's ravages. Due in part to organic changes in the brain, and abetted by self-denigration, depression sufferers are led to twist the facts to conform to their distorted version of reality. When those neurotransmitters stopped doing their job, they set in motion a mindset primed for denial. The odds of overcoming it depend upon an empathetic grasp of their version of the truth. Mental health professionals call this "getting into your partner's head."

The dictionary definition of empathy is "the intellectual identification with or vicarious experiencing of the feelings, thoughts, or attitudes of another." While it is not possible for the non-depressed to experience the feelings of depression, fallout partners should accept that their mates are telling the truth as they see it. The depressed "know" they are doing nothing wrong and have expressed their thoughts in crystal-clear fashion. The better able you are to grasp their conviction of blamelessness, the better you will understand why they are so ready to blame others. To you, your partner's denial of depression as the source of his or her negative assessment of the marriage is misguided and selfish; to your partner, you are the one in denial. The sender of the E-mail, "I am very bitter and I quit," believed he had made himself clear and so felt justified in instructing his wife not to communicate again.

Although a cool, scientific rationale does help explain the oddities of depressed behavior—confused thinking, hopelessness, resentment and anger, withdrawal from intimacy—an empathetic alternative is to note how similar are depression and depression fallout. Fallout partners are at first confused about the tremors shaking the relationship; after a period of self-blame, they shift blame to their mates; they lose self-esteem and become demoralized; then they grow resentful and angry; eventually, even if still in love, they long to terminate the union. Viewed in this manner, depression and depression fallout follow the same curve. Think of the two states of mind as eerie doppelgängers that are separated only by their genesis. While you are demoralized because of real-life events and your partner is depressed because of brain chemistry, you both experience feelings of helplessness and hopelessness. Your advantage is that somewhere in the five fallout stages, you accurately identify the role of your partner's depression in shaping your feelings and reactions. Your partner, unable to do the same, falls back on denial and blames you.

You also have the advantage of being able to reason logically and to control or moderate your emotions. Your depressed partner's emotional fuse is clipped so short that small aggravations set off volcanic eruptions, which in turn ignite your own. This negative chain reaction will be evident if you try to imagine your part in a scene that opens with a wife's assertion that her husband is depressed. The wife has boned up on depression and believes she will take command of the conversation and direct it to its logical conclusion. But when her mate derisively snaps back, "What me, depressed? If anyone's depressed around here, it's you," she retorts that that is a preposterous statement; both partners are now cross and no progress has been made. Her intention to explain that one in every five people suffers from depression goes into the ditch, and depression is now a hot-button issue. The wife's second attempt to propose medication is met with the accusation that she is undermining their marriage. She leaves the room without answering because her husband's accusation now strikes her as plausible; she decides to make a big effort to be a more loving and supportive partner.

After additional unsuccessful attempts to overcome her partner's denial that he is depressed, the wife has stored up a truckload of what she believes to be fully warranted resentments. She sets to collecting evidence for her "case" against him—his condescension, his hurtful accusations—and sees him as the primary obstacle to a guilt-free, happy future. After months of secretly mulling this over, she wishes her husband would suggest a divorce because that would allow her to move on to a relatively guilt-free, contented life without him. This example of the doppelgänger phenomenon should help you muster some empathy for your depressed partner—a valuable tool in overcoming denial—and also point out the danger of losing your cool. If your persuasive arts still need help, take a lesson from the science of marketing.

## Persuasion As the Science of Marketing

While waiting for a dentist appointment, I leafed through a copy of *Scientific American* and came across an article entitled "The Science of Persuasion." Across the top ran the headline: "Salespeople, politicians, friends and family all have a stake in getting you to agree to their requests. Social psychology has determined the basic principles that govern getting to 'yes.'" The author, Robert B. Cialdini, Regents' Professor of Psychology at Arizona State University, opens with a spoof on those "Hello there" letters that trick us into buying something we don't want or contributing to a cause we aren't interested in, and then lays out the six basic ingredients of a successful marketing campaign: reciprocity ("If you do this, I'll do that"); consistency (the buyer's desire to be, and to appear, consistent); social validation (demonstrating, or merely implying, that others just like us have already complied; liking (people prefer to say yes to those they like); authority ("Four out of five doctors recommend our product"); and scarcity ("Limited time to accept this offer").

Selling depression to a reluctant buyer is harder than selling a magazine subscription, but the same principles apply. In lieu of a discount coupon, offer to stop worrying about your partner's mental health for a set period; promise that you, too, will go see your doctor; be endlessly proud and grateful for compliance with your wishes; or do whatever you think will be most enticing. Cialdini introduces consistency with the example of one small change made in a restaurant's reservations policy that dramatically reduced the number of no-show patrons. Instead of saying, "Please call if you have to change your plans," the table booker asked patrons, "Will you please call if you have to change your plans?" and politely paused and waited for a response. By gently forcing a commitment on the part of your partner, you make backing out more difficult and preempt any complaints of nagging and harping if a second or third (subtle) arm-twisting session is required.

For social validation of depression, Cialdini recommends going for quality rather than quantity. Cull that long list of the rich, talented, and famous high achievers and cite those who will resonate with your partner. Leave mass-market figures, like the nineteen million Americans who suffer from this illness, aside. Instead, try sharing the news that a niece or nephew (or friend, coworker, or neighbor), or the investment banker who at thirty-three has retired to the Bahamas, has been on Prozac for years.

As to the marketing ingredient called "liking," even though not currently on display, your partner both likes and loves you, and has surely relied on your advice in the past. Still, taking care to look your best when you launch your campaign can tilt the outcome in your favor. When the American Heart Association began hiring attractive fund-raisers, it noted quickly that they generated nearly twice as many donations as the persuasive but less eye-catching ones. If your wife always notices when your shoes aren't shined and your hair is too long, get a haircut and some shoe polish; if your husband loves you in that blue dress and with your hair unbound, do the necessary in preparation for the discussion.

Projecting authority depends on a sure command of the facts: Depression is an illness, not a state of mind; depression often travels from one generation to another (let the "blame" fall on a parent or grandparent rather than the individual); no one in the world is capable of controlling their neurotransmitters; all the studies show that antidepressants do work; and so forth. The final marketing rule, perceived scarcity of the product, won't sell your argument, but a subrule of scarcity will: the limited time offer. "Buy this product [your advice] now, because if you don't . . ." may sound as though you are making a threat, but in fallout idiom this is called setting boundaries. The why, when, and how of boundary setting, and other fallout strategies, are next on the agenda.

# 4

# Drawing a Line
# in the Sand

Families and couples are more than the sum of their parts. The most successful and mutually gratifying relationships are those in which the members pull together and honor collectively established rules and behavioral boundaries. When people know what is expected of them, and what can be expected from others, they feel grounded and secure, an integral part of a web that fosters mutual trust and protects against adversity. Spinning the web as a team is a reminder of shared goals, and of the benefits of cooperation and a healthy sense of interdependence. Behaving predictably and respecting the feelings of others is mutually gratifying to all concerned and helps the family or couple to grow closer and to prosper. But depression exempts itself from these governing rules. Instead of bending to them, it makes up its own rules, changes them from minute to minute, breaks agreements spoken and unspoken, shatters expectations, and injects chaos into the family unit.

Accepting the imperatives of depression's rules provides

some protection from the hurtful assault upon your feelings, but depersonalizing behavior by attributing its cause to an illness does not imply it should be excused and allowed to run rampant. Like all bad behavior, that driven by depression can and should be controlled by setting boundaries to limit it. And while depression sufferers are marching to a different and very insistent drummer, they are neither stupid nor unable to control themselves. Indeed, they supply maddening evidence of this by behaving normally when out and about with others, then reverting abruptly to unacceptable ways as soon as you are alone together. Someone has to inject order or the relationship will crumble. Unless the fallout partner takes on this task, the rules of depression will prevail by default.

This chapter has three objectives, the first of which is to prove to you that no matter how outlandish your partner's behavior seems to you, other fallout mates have witnessed the same. As one Board poster observed, every inch of the Twilight Zone has been mapped before you entered it. The second objective is to give you another close look at how depression works its black magic. Once you see the sleight of hand involved, you will be less easily manipulated into believing that what you witness is the whole truth. The third objective is to show how you can draw some lines in the sand that your partner cannot easily cross and to arm you with counterstrategies of your own.

## CASTING THE "IT" AS VILLAIN

Neurobiologist Oliver Sacks has observed that "Any disease introduces a doubleness into life—an 'it,' with all its own needs, demands, and limitations." Depression is the "it" in your relationship, an uninvited and unruly guest who eventually must be tamed by treatment. In the interim, you need to acknowledge and learn how to live with its presence without trading in your integrity and sense of self.

All men and women in a relationship with a depressed spouse or lover wonder where the person they fell in love with has gone. They catch reassuring glimpses of their true beloved in fleeting moments of mutual tenderness and trust, only to come face-to-face again with their "new" partner, who seems intent on doling out confusion, hurtful criticism, and behavior designed to annoy and enrage. Predictably, fallout partners come to interpret such treatment as calculated acts of meanness, or as evidence of their partners' true feelings for them. Nothing could be further from the truth. Depression, not your husband, wife, or lover, is the real villain in this scenario and your mate's behavior, far from being calculated, is governed by the illness.

Emotional abuse is hard to define. For those spared experience of it, the term conjures up major shouting matches and insults tossed like grenades, but the impact of subtler slights on the ego is cumulative. What seems at the moment a relatively minor infraction of conduct, not worth the risk of a confrontational scene, will dig in and expand unless fallout partners recognize it as part of a larger pattern that does deserve the name of emotional abuse. Moderating the hurtful behavior of the depressed is far more difficult than teaching good manners to children. It's wise to remember at all times that you are dealing with an adult.

Punishment in the traditional sense will exacerbate rather than control the behavior and will fortify your partner's conviction that you do not understand or care about his or her inner pain. Ultimatums can be dangerous; what you say and what your partner hears may be quite different.

Boundaries that take into account the feelings that drive the unwanted behavior are the most effective, so further delving into your partner's mind is in order.

## DR. JEKYLL AND MR. OR MS. HYDE

Whether perpetrated by the long or newly married, the corporate lawyer or the supermarket clerk, the uniformity of depressive behavior is striking. Contrary to the belief of many psychotherapists and psychiatrists, Message Board evidence strongly suggests that depressed men and women, in the privacy of their own homes, read from the same script. Some depressed women are indeed more ruminative, churning their internal misery in isolated silence like reclusive Greta Garbos. Some depressed men do adopt a more angry and aggressive attitude, and self-medicate with alcohol and work. But judging by the approximately fifteen thousand posts registered to date on the Message Board, and by a steady flow of agonized E-mails received from fallout readers, both sexes follow the same discernible patterns, often switching between feminine and masculine styles as they ride the depression roller coaster.

Consider, for instance, the charming Dr. Jekyll and the dreadful Mr. (or Ms.) Hyde who live together inside every depressed person. Mr. Hyde drags himself off the sofa where he has spent his Saturday and heads for the bathroom, muttering that he's damned if he wants to spend the evening with your boring friends—they are always your friends, not his—and that he had planned to clean the garage/write a report for a meeting/play with the kids/do all the chores you've harped about all day. Dressed and ready at last, Mr. Hyde casts furtive glances at you, shaking his head as if in astonishment and uttering little grunts easily translated as "I can't believe it." You ask what's the matter; he, enunciating every syllable as though you were a halfwit, asks why on earth you decided to put on that dress/parted your hair in the middle/forgot to put in your contact lenses. Having dented your self-esteem, he whacks away at it during the drive over, complaining about the bad mood you were in some day last week/your failure to put gas in the car/the president you personally elected by casting your vote for the wrong party. The hammering continues right up to the moment that your host opens the front door.

"Hi!" says Dr. Jekyll with evident enthusiasm. He bounds from guest to guest, bussing cheeks and slapping shoulders as he heads for the bar. "What would you like, sweetie?" he asks, swinging his arm around your waist and giving a little squeeze. "Wow, you look great!" he tells the hostess. "If I didn't have such a gorgeous wife"—he turns a loving eye on you—"I'd be jealous. Are we lucky, or what?" he says to the host, chuckling like a child being tickled. Dr. Jekyll is a bon vivant, the life of the party, the loving spouse who exudes charm and bonhomie. During the buffet dinner (he has chosen a seat on the opposite side of the room), you note that he listens attentively to those he is with, nods alertly while they talk, and appears responsive. Occasionally, he seeks out your eye and twinkles to let his companions know how truly adorable and cherished you are. Little bursts of laughter emanate from his corner, and you imagine the conversations between couples later in the evening: "Aren't the Jekylls fun? Isn't he just divine?"

You ride home with Mr. Hyde, whose evening you have ruined. "What were those baleful looks you kept giving me? You could at least pretend to have a good time instead of treating me like I'm Caligula." Delivering a final parting shot—"And you claim I'm the one who's depressed!"—Mr. Hyde throws himself on the sofa, turns on the television, and says he doesn't feel like coming to bed. Exhausted by seething or crying, you fall asleep alone.

The advice that you control your temper and say nothing sounds heartless, but imagine the conversation that would take place if you complained bitterly of having been mistreated. The most probable comeback would be that you are always nagging him to talk instead of sulking silently, so why are you now berating him for being cheerful and having fun, and that he went out of his way to compliment you in front of the other guests, and you just glowered, and on and on. Instead, try to let go of the incident until you have a better grasp of what you can tolerate and what deserves a boundary.

The Jekyll-Hyde tale has been so often recounted on the Message Board that new versions of it draw been-there-done-that responses. Colin's opens with a verbatim account of his depressed wife's diatribe three months after having been prescribed an antidepressant dose so low it couldn't cheer up a hamster. "I'm done pretending," she announced thirty minutes before a dozen mothers and children arrived for their son's fourth birthday party. "I don't love you and I never will." Colin says he was such a basket case as a result that he remembers almost nothing of the party other than how "happy and cheerful she was, blah, blah, blah." It would be easy to view his wife as a brave mother rising above her distress in order to spare the kids had she not reverted to Ms. Hyde—"Thank God they've gone, I'm going to bed"—as soon as the last guest left, leaving Colin to comfort their son and put him to bed. "I can take it when she dumps on me," says Colin, "but what am I supposed to do when she pulls this stuff in front of our child?" The answer is, set a boundary: no conflict in front of the kids, their well-being comes first.

Louisa's version involves a similarly startling assessment of their marriage by Mr. Hyde that was interrupted by a phone call, taken by Dr. Jekyll. In a tone full of lively enthusiasm he chatted at length with a favorite uncle about fly-fishing and football games as though the happiest of men and, on hanging up, resumed his diatribe. "It amazes me how grumpy and argumentative my wife is with me and how great with friends and colleagues," chimes in Phil. "The phone rings and her face changes and she morphs into some happy person. The minute she hangs up, Sad Sack is back."

These shifts *are* amazing, but although they may upset

you, they are rarely deliberately designed to be hurtful. With the exception of Colin's story, which involved a child, escalating them into a big deal isn't a practical solution. You cannot control the way a depressed person feels. Your aim is to try to control the consequences of his or her feelings, and that in turn means differentiating between the annoying and the intolerable. If your partner's internal feelings are externalized as, for instance, behavior that threatens a child's emotional stability, it's time to set a boundary. Out-of-control drinking and drugging also call for boundaries because they endanger the welfare of others. If you are constantly railed at and criticized to the point of feeling demoralized and helpless, stand up for yourself by drawing a line in the sand, but be specific; complaining in generalities won't work.

The Jekyll-Hyde dualism isn't some calculated plot to deceive; we depression sufferers use it to hide our frailties and vulnerability from the eyes of outsiders (and sometimes from ourselves) and to maintain our dignity. Single at the time, I hurt no one but myself when, at the close of days made tolerable by a job I loved, I lay spread-eagled on the bed and stared at the ceiling while contemplating suicide disguised as accident, to spare my daughter pain. If the phone rang, I swung into animated action, regretfully declining an invitation to the movies because I had just a moment before made another date. On hanging up, I worried that if I died, no one would come to my funeral, yet the next day acted in the office as though my only concern was getting the job done well. When your depressed partner puts on the Jekyll mask, try to remember that its purpose is to keep the world from knowing how weak and miserable she is. Remember, too, that she is terrified of being pitied and truly believes that no one really understands her, and wouldn't like her if they did. A kinder description of the Jekyll mask is coping mechanism, but holding up this jolly persona takes enormous energy. A few hours spent dining with friends or playing the cheerful mom at a birthday party is exhausting; when the front door closes, depressives let the pretense crash and burn.

For this, too, your partner has reasons: Alone with you, he feels safe unmasked. He knows you love him, and that you will not discard him as an acquaintance might; he knows you will not fire or demote him, and counts on you not to complain about him to your friends or family. This contorted but deeply rooted trust in the devotion and patience of an intimate is an extreme version of wandering around the house without makeup or a shave. From the fallout perspective, however, it looks like one of a barrage of attacks on your self-esteem, a determined campaign to undermine, disparage, and reduce you to the status of a non-person.

## ZIGZAGS AND NON SEQUITURS

As bewildering as the mask exchange is the ability to turn on a dime. Depression sufferers are unpredictable and illogical; these are symptoms of the illness. Conversations about what time to have dinner or which video to rent turn into a rant against in-laws or a door-slamming departure from the room. Inquire if they had a good day at the office and you may be treated to an indictment that begins with your faults and ends with threats of suicide. As Maggie Mae puts it, "Whenever I ask my depressed husband how he's going to spend the weekend, first he sulks as though I had cornered him and then he massages his anger by attacking me personally." She knows the rampage is finally over when his outrage turns to the American political system because "that's my cue that he has finally cleaned out his liver, and that life will be somewhat peaceable for a while."

Fallout stories like these unravel the interconnected web that partners rely on as both safety net and security blanket. Non-depressed mates, blindsided by unpredictable behavior and shifting feelings that seem to come from nowhere, take a misstep in trying to connect them to reality. A basic boundary rule for them is not to engage and not to take everything as a personal insult. Equally important, never argue on depression's terms; leave the room and add (without sarcasm if you can) that you are sorry he or she is feeling down today. That's hard, but it's doable; it will save you a great deal of useless grief and will have a positive rather than negative impact on your partner.

From a depressed perspective, the scales of justice are always out of kilter; eventually, fallouts adopt the same viewpoint. Weighing the small favors and accommodations exchanged in every partnership, each finds the balance tipped in the other's favor. Jade's husband of eleven years, who lays claim to a midlife crisis at age thirty-five, expects her to conform to his new self-imposed routine. "We used to be a close family," she says, "but nowadays he sneaks in the door, no hello, no eye contact, and heads for the computer. When the kids and I sit down for dinner he says he's not hungry, but the food is gone in the morning." One night Jade got so mad that she threw his dinner out instead of leaving it for him, and he transferred guilt to Jade by saying that she was trying to starve him out of the house. Twice a week on average, Jason's depressed wife calls him at the office because her car has died on the way to the market or the children's school. When he tells her for the umpteenth time to get it fixed, she goes into a super-aggrieved routine: "Oh, so you think you're doing me a big favor. Well, don't worry, I'll never ask you for a favor again." And then, says Jason, she "complains about how awful her life is and how it's not her fault we don't have the money to buy a house or a nice new car, or even enough to fix this one, and besides she can't find her credit card (again), and she has no time to go get the car fixed because I insisted she join my family for vacation so she has no vacation time to spare."

As one poster expressed it, trying to have a close relationship with a depressed person is like walking through a minefield. Erica says she is never thanked when she tries to adapt to her husband's moods and to offer encouragement; her husband's view is that he is the one handing out heavy-duty support to her. "Worst of all are the reprieve times that lead me to believe that everything will finally be all right again," Erica adds. "They throw me off balance more than anything he does." Over time, the accumulation of hurts inhibits fallout sufferers from offering the supportive words and gestures that are as necessary to a depressive as good professional treatment. One fallout husband headed his post "End of Rope," and described "the living hell that is private and silent, about which the world knows nothing. It's like fighting with a giant beast in a small room," a message that could have been written by a depression war correspondent.

While many specific transgressions practiced by depressed partners can be contained when boundaries are set, there is virtually no way to stop this generalized behavior dead in its tracks. The masks, the zigzags and non sequiturs, and the self-pity of the depressed are all implacable fixtures of depression. In *Undoing Depression*, a book written for his fellow depression sufferers, Richard O'Connor explains why.

## WHEN MOOD CHANGES TAKE THE PLACE OF EMOTIONS

Depression sufferers who wonder what's the matter with them must first heave a sigh of relief on reading *Undoing Depression* and then gawk in surprise when they hear the author's answer to why it is so hard for them to change. A psychotherapist who has long battled his own depression and understands its exigencies, Richard O'Connor identifies with the absence of feeling we experience, a void created in part by a fear of emotions we cannot control. "Instead of the normal fluctuations of happiness, sadness, disappointment, joy, desire, and anger that most people cycle through many times a day," he writes, "depressed people feel a kind of gray neutrality that translates into subterranean tectonic shifts in mood."

What depressed persons typically experience are mood changes rather than emotions. One minute the sun is shining, and then without warning, and without our knowing why, it is in eclipse, and we are sad, down, discouraged, and devoid of energy. Although these whiplashing mood shifts seem to come out of the blue, they are caused, O'Connor explains, by an unfelt feeling related to some interpersonal event. "Something happens that makes us angry, makes us feel hurt, sad, or scared—or even happy—but the event doesn't register on our consciousness. The feeling seems disconnected from reality; we don't understand what's going on in ourselves so we feel inadequate, out of control, frustrated—depressed again."

So far, so good, but then comes a rude awakening from the indulgent conviction that somehow our feelings and behavior are justified by the fact that we are at the mercy of those tectonic shifts in mood. This is not so, says O'Connor. He believes that the major reason why people with depression—even those who are on medication and in therapy and enjoy the support of their intimates—go on behaving in self-destructive ways is that they are simply unable to imagine an alternative. "We know how to do depression. We are experts at it. Our feelings about ourselves and the way we see the world have forced us over the years to develop a very special set of skills" in a vain effort to save ourselves pain. Expecting us to stop being depressed is like expecting a blind person to suddenly see, "with one important difference; eventually, we can do it."

O'Connor's unorthodox view of change and recovery is a strong argument for boundary setting by fallout partners, not as a punitive attempt to extract compliance, but as a firm and helpful reminder that the "habit" of being and acting depressed can be broken. His description of our sense of "estrangement from the world, our noses pushed up against the glass watching real life go on behind the window, and a consequent bitterness, hurt, or resentment" takes hold in our psyches like a fish hook. The unfairness of it all justifies our anger. Giving in to the anger can be, as O'Connor puts it, "so heady [and] tempting, can make us feel so good, that we indulge ourselves in carrying the fight forward till our opponent is humiliated." The once-familiar comforts of love and affection, even when offered by a dearly loved spouse or child, now fail to touch us, blocked as they are by our emotionally frozen state. Our assumption that everyone else is happy most of the time, and that there is something wrong with us for not feeling the same way, is a learned state of mind that can be replaced with a more positive and rewarding one.

If Richard O'Connor has an Old Ramblings box, I suspect it contains jotted notations, many of them written with the help of alcohol, that closely resemble my own. "*Cogito, ergo sum*—okay, but who exactly am I? To be is hardly enough. Surely I must be someone." Lists of attributes I admired in my friends, and then, "I have none of these." "I feel zero—zero to begin, zero in the middle, zero to the end." "My 'self' is just a button pushed by others. I am a creature of them, not me. I take my cues and clues as to my existence from them, and am thus not in my own control, only at their disposal. What will happen if they choose to dispose of me?" "When I look up, I see chaos;

others see light." "It's astounding to hear other people talk about their objectives and goals. Mine have to do with staying alive." More than fifteen years and some ten thousand antidepressant pills later, turning these "facts" into fiction is still a wrestling match between me and my depression.

Such is the mind of a depressed person. Keeping it afloat demands so much vigilance and energy that we are dumbfounded by a partner's failure to intuit our inner pain and self-disgust. Desperate to attract attention, and torn between parading naked and preserving our facade, we alternately invite and resent signs of sympathy and support. Asked how we feel, we retreat into hurt silence or shout about our pain. The manipulative scenes we manufacture are often staged to gain attention and to reassure ourselves that we count for something in this world. When a spouse or lover turns away or chastises us for thoughtless behavior, we feel utterly betrayed, unloved, and alone. In fact, we feel remarkably like our fallout partners do. It is ironic that depression sufferers and fallout sufferers use the same similes; we are all of us riding roller coasters, walking on eggshells, battling with the same large beast in the same small room.

## BOUNDARY SETTING, STAGE ONE: FIRST THINGS FIRST

Fallout partners, understandably leery of instigating a shouting match that will leave them emotionally depleted and hostile, should review the foregoing section before every boundary discussion and use its precepts in tandem with your right to fair treatment from the person you love.

Keep previous successes and mishaps in mind as a guide. If you have inadvertently pushed some panic and anger buttons in the past, steer clear of them this time. Stick to a prepared agenda, use diplomatic language, and don't rely on children or other family and friends as buffers; the business between you is private and airing it in front of others is verboten. Most important of all, use what you now know about a depressed person's mind; do not expect it to work like yours, nor to react predictably to the same stimuli. Your tears may well serve to deepen your spouse's sense of unworthiness and his inability to experience or give happiness; your anger may reinforce her accusation that you, not depression, are the cause of her unhappiness. If there is an explosion or a deadlocked silence, say you sympathize with their distress and that you will wait in another room until they feel ready to resume the conversation; alternatively, ask if they will please set a time of their choosing, and say that you know you can count on them to keep their word.

Sentences opened by "You always" or "You never" strike an accusatory chord; a better strategy is to focus on your feelings and to introduce them by saying "I." Be explicit in expressing how you feel: invisible when your partner walks in the door without saying hello; hurt when he or she flinches at an affectionate gesture; no longer loved or lovable when he or she opts for the sofa instead of your bed. Invite your mate to do the same and listen without interrupting, bearing in mind how painfully difficult it is for the depressed to describe their internal landscape. Two sets of feelings on the table present opportunities for agreement: We love each other; we share the same prob lem; we need to find mutually agreed-upon solutions.

## BOUNDARY SETTING, STAGE TWO: MAKING CHOICES

The boundaries selected should take into account the interactive pattern of the relationship before the illness settled in. Depression creates so many problems that fall-out partners are in danger of confusing new behavioral lapses with old ones that preexisted the illness. In every healthy relationship, each member learns to accommo-date the personal idiosyncrasies of the other. Although they may not like this or that habit, they accept that nobody's perfect. If a spouse has always spent an hour on her computer after dinner, her wish to an hour more is an easy accommodation to make and will rank low on her husband's list. If a live-in lover is chronically recalcitrant about sharing chores, making a federal case about his recent failure to take out the garbage is a waste of time and ammunition. Use as a yardstick what you can and cannot tolerate in the present scheme of things.

A good approach to selecting boundaries is to make a list of everything new your partner does that drives you crazy and then winnow it down to a few depression-related biggies. A typical list before editing might include the following:

1. Say good morning when you wake up and greet me civilly each evening.

2. Stop acting like an adolescent; you're supposed to be a grown-up.

3. Eat with the rest of the family.

4. Never argue in front of the kids.

5. Quit laying your anger on me.

6. Never use breaking up with me as a threat.

7. Stop blaming me for everything.

8. Sleep in the bedroom, not on the couch.

9. Don't spend all night on the computer or watching television.

10. Keep your promises.

11. Do your assigned chores.

12. No insults allowed.

13. Stop drinking.

14. No threatening gestures.

15. No violence, whether directed at me or inanimate objects.

You don't have to consult with a psychologist or marriage counselor to figure out which boundaries will register with your partner or to select those he or she is able to comply with right now. Some, such as "Quit laying your anger on me" and "Stop blaming me for everything," are guaranteed to jump-start the kind of behavior you had hoped to avoid. Others—"Keep your promises," for example—are too vague to make much of an impact. When bargaining with someone who is depressed, specificity is paramount. "Please" works better than naked imperatives: "Please say good morning" or "Please eat with the family so the kids won't worry."

An edited list might be winnowed down to four items: "No arguing or angry displays in front of the children"; "When you make a specific promise to do something, please follow through"; "Treat me with courtesy and civility when we are alone"; and "No threats of violence of any kind." Any of the most important items you choose—a ban on insults, threats, and violence—must carry a penalty, an explicit "If you do this, I will . . ." without which compliance is unlikely.

## BOUNDARY SETTING, STAGE THREE: DRAWING LINES THAT CAN RESIST THE INCOMING TIDE

The purpose of boundaries is to make everyone feel less hassled and more secure, so to be effective they must be negotiated by both parties and have agreed-upon consequences—an "or else" on which you are prepared to act. Fallouts typically complain that depressed mates can't concentrate for more than sixty seconds, but dysfunctional neurotransmitters do not mysteriously tinker with innate intelligence. Although your partner does think irrationally, he or she is capable of moderating both speech and behavior, providing the requests made are within their power to honor; instructions to lighten up and think positive might as well be issued in Chinese. If you leave the room instead of retaliating every time an insult is hurled, your partner will get the message and after a time start putting a lid on verbal abuse. Engaging in the fray is self-defeating and demoralizing because you are really arguing with an illness, and there is little doubt about who will be the winner.

Instead of saying "I hate it when you sit in front of your computer looking at porn/E-mailing Internet boyfriends/playing the same game ad infinitum," suggest three hours as a maximum and only after the dishes are done and the children are in bed. The "or else" might be that if your mate exceeds the limit you will turn off the computer yourself, in spite of the fact that you realize it will make him or her feel like a child. You cannot order your spouse to sleep in the same room with you, but you can put sheets and a blanket on the sofa or spare bed, offer a good-night kiss, and move the television to the bedroom. If you want the daily chores done, list all of them, check off those you will do yourself, and warn that the remaining ones—picking up the laundered shirts, paying the electric bill, filling the antiallergy prescription—will otherwise go undone. For items such as clearing out the garage or putting up shelves in the living room, get estimates and explain that unless your beloved knuckles down you will ask his best friend to take on the job or, money permitting, you will use housekeeping or family-entertainment funds to pay their cost.

Deliberately shaming your depressed partner into positive action seems cruel, but conquering the self-defeating habits typical of depression can actually strengthen his or her wilted self-esteem. Bowing to the reality of those tectonic shifts of mood, it is wise to extend a ban on arguments in front of the children to include no snapping at the kids as well. (You might suggest that when your spouse feels like doing that, he or she should run around the block or shout alone in the garage.) The "or else" depends on how often it happens after the boundary has been drawn; multiple breaches might necessitate telling your partner that you intend to ask the children's teachers to be on the alert for possible classroom behavioral problems due to family conflict, a well-documented consequence for offspring of a depressed parent.

## HANDLING PHYSICAL VIOLENCE

The inchoate anger bred by depression can rise to such an intolerable level that it spins out of control and manifests itself in physical violence. In *The Noonday Demon: An Atlas of Depression,* author Andrew Solomon recounts a serious falling-out with a lover who had betrayed him. "I attacked him with a ferocity unlike any I had experienced before, threw him against a wall, and socked him repeatedly, breaking both his jaw and his nose," he writes. "I felt as though I were disappearing, and somewhere deep in the most primitive part of my brain, I felt that violence was the only way I could keep my self and mind in the world." "It took," says Solomon, "a powerful summoning of my superego to save me from strangling him."

Tragedy is not always averted. In June 2001, a Texan

wife and mother who had suffered from postpartum depression following the birth of each of her five children drowned them one by one in the bathtub, then quietly gave herself up to the police. Although at no previous time had Andrea Yates threatened to harm her offspring, after the fourth was born she twice tried to kill herself and was prescribed antidepressants and an antipsychotic, Haldol, which treats symptoms like hallucinations, delusions, paranoia, and deeply confused thinking. For some reason, her doctor discontinued this medication a short while before the murders occurred, thus perhaps removing a barrier against her impulses. According to media reports, she had been contemplating the murders for some time.

Although extreme and terrifying events such as these are rare, they are a crimson warning that minor acts of violence may presage major ones. In my first book I chronicled a severely depressed adolescent's progression from breaking plates against the wall to hurling them at her mother, and told as well the story of a woman whose depressed lover threatened her with scissors during an argument, then locked her out of the house. While the Message Board does not often report tales of violence, the topic does arise. One example was Agate's frightened post about her depressed husband's sudden shift from verbal to physical abuse: "My pleading with him to see a doctor tripped him into one of his rages and he flung me against the wall. I am totally shell-shocked," she writes. "This is not the husband I once knew."

If physically threatened, leave the house immediately

and call your partner's doctor and psychotherapist for advice before returning. Should he or she not have one, call 911, if only to shock your mate into realizing that the illness has the upper hand. This is a painful step to take, often wrongly interpreted by fallouts as a betrayal, but violence feeds on itself. No matter how genuinely apologetic and appalled the depressed partner may be after the fact, he or she needs more than your love and support.

Several replies to Agate's message tied relatively minor violence—pushing, shoving, gripping an arm hard enough to hurt—to the non-depressed lover's own loss of temper. "We would be having tense, angry words and I would unconsciously ball my fists and start punctuating my remarks with them, getting into his personal space and glaring eye to eye," writes Cynthia, "and then my safety valve would kick in and I would throw up my hands and say, 'I'm outta here. This is ridiculous. We're getting nowhere.' And that's when it would happen, just as I was gathering up my things and walking toward the door." Cynthia's point is that she was a participant in the ratcheting-up of her lover's temper, and that by moderating her own temper, she learned she could reduce the possibility that things might get physical. But the real lesson to be learned from her post is that depression can dismantle that safety valve.

I am not suggesting that fallouts call the police every time their partners slam a door or kick a chair. I am advising caution, concern, and a demand, backed up by an "or else," that medical and psychotherapeutic help be sought.

# EXPRESSING EMOTIONAL NEEDS:
# A SUCCESS STORY

Some Message Board diplomats favor a "needs" list to express what they must have to keep their emotional clock ticking. When I asked posters to provide examples of these needs, one flagged a pitfall of all such requests: voicing them too late. "I think most fallouts wait until the situation is so crazy and out of control that we can't live with it any longer," Purple replied. "The treatment we're subjected to does such a number on our self-esteem that we lose confidence in our ability to control it. By the time I presented my needs list, I saw separation as my only option. In hindsight, I should have been a lot tougher much earlier." A Board veteran who has chalked up 641 posts that lead to a happy ending, Purple wisely chose to put on paper what she wanted to tell her husband:

1. I need you to respect my feelings. Ignoring Mother's Day was a terrible slap in the face and left me feeling unloved and unappreciated as both wife and mother of our child. When you stay out late without calling or ditch plans we've made together, I worry and get upset. Telling me you're a big boy and can take care of yourself is the equivalent of ignoring my concerns.

2. I need friendship. Friends confide in one another, they laugh, they cry, they share things and enjoy being together. I miss out on all that because our daily life is always centered on you, not on us.

3. I need communication and openness about our current financial state and our plans for the future. That means planning together, not buying whatever you feel like buying without consultation.

4. [Which Purple calls "the biggie"] I need honesty. You call the dodging and backtracking white lies, like skipping your therapy appointment and telling me you went, but if I can't trust you with little things, then how can I trust you with big ones?

In the conversation that followed, Purple's husband said that although he understood her needs and considered them reasonable, it was too difficult to meet them and the demands of his professional life as well. Purple packed her suitcases on the spot, scooped up their six-year-old, and moved to her mother's house for two weeks to give him time to reconsider. In frequent phone calls back and forth, she backed up her list with more specifics and added a critical boundary: "Never denigrate or unjustly criticize me in front of our daughter. She learns from what she sees and lives with daily. When you say you're not sure you want to be married anymore and that I am the cause of your unhappiness, you are instilling in her a very distorted idea of what constitutes love." Conditions for a return home included observance of Purple's needs and boundaries, his admission that he was depressed and that he make without delay an appointment with a psychiatrist, as well as his agreement to start psychotherapy to rediscover the loving husband he once had been.

"I'm not sure what the magic words were," Purple wound up, "perhaps being clear that if he liked himself the way he was he would have to go it alone, or perhaps my final message: 'We've tried it your way. Now I'd like you to try it my way.'" Had I been in her depressed husband's shoes, the fact that Purple had done her depression home-work, that she recognized that compliance wouldn't be easy for him, and that she promised to be patient and sup-portive for as long as he kept his part of the bargain would have been key factors in strengthening my resolve to suc-ceed. The bargain worked; a year later, says Purple, they are following "a completely different scenario. My husband has learned to monitor and control his moods instead of giving in to them. He faithfully takes his antidepressants and turns up on time for his doctor and therapy appoint-ments. Talking about depression isn't taboo anymore. We're pretty much back to normal and very happy."

## A WRAP-UP OF PITFALLS AND HOW TO SIDESTEP THEM

A major pitfall, as noted, is procrastination. The behavior that accompanies depression is so unexpected and puz-zling that non-depressed partners avert their eyes in the hope they are witnessing a temporary departure from the norm. Accumulated hurts and growing resentment are bottled up until the cork pops and angry fizz bubbles out. As do many fallout sufferers, Chey allowed months to pass in stoic silence; only when her emotions had reached overload did she give raucous voice to them, not in the form of boundaries subject to negotiation but as enraged ultimatums with little chance of success. When fallouts give way to tears, tantrums, and trading accusations, they abdicate control, and the deceptive calm that follows such scenes lulls them into thinking that the crisis has past. These "reprieve times," during which life appears normal once again, drain the reservoir of hope. "Just when I think I've made an impact," says Chey, "the same thing happens again, leaving me even more frustrated, disappointed, and let down than before." As hope dwindles, so do the odds that the relationship will survive.

Fear of angry confrontation is one reason for procrastination; another is excessive concern for the fragility of the depressive mindset. Ginger, a social worker who is knowledgeable about this illness and one of the wisest Message Board posters, admits she never presented her depressed husband with carefully prepared lists and demands. "I knew he was sick and unable to think clearly, so I cut him a lot of slack and put up with repeated bad behavior." Instead, she mounted a campaign to get her husband back on the antidepressants he had abandoned. "As long as I had a plan, an overriding goal that would solve all our problems, I felt able to cope with the situation," she explains. But sure enough, eventually the cork popped, not during a head-to-head battle, but when her husband chose to linger at the boss's Halloween party instead of trick or treating with Ginger and the kids as promised. Once the limits of emotional endurance are breached, opting out of the relationship can seem the only way to preserve one's inner unity. Soon after the seemingly minor incident, Ginger asked for a divorce.

Jersey, a fallout husband and the father of a Down syndrome child who "needs a little extra help to stay even in life," says that he and his wife have successfully encouraged their son to observe the same family rules that govern their other child. "If he can do it, why can't my wife?" Perhaps it is because Jersey has never explicitly insisted she do so, or perhaps he has fallen into the dangerous habit of trying continually to adjust to his wife's ephemeral mood changes, mistaking them for bona fide emotions. Whichever the case, Tim's countercomment on boundaries and needs is pertinent: "I think a better word than boundaries is 'responsibilities,'" he writes. "Sick or not, depressives are adults and must accept that their actions have consequences. We all make decisions every day, but we take into account how they will affect others before choosing a course of action. My approach is to ask my wife to spend more time thinking about her choices, not just barging ahead and doing whatever she feels like. Depression is an illness—not an excuse."

Another potential pitfall is lack of specificity in making demands and failing to follow through on the "or else." Instead of a short, tidy list, Just Me wrote down twenty heartfelt but muddled needs and wants, ran a bath for her husband, and taped it above the tub. "I guess he couldn't get his mind around such a huge inventory so it ended up antagonizing him," she says in retrospect. "The only use he put it to was to point out that I wasn't doing for him what I claimed I needed him to do for me." Jenna, whose live-in boyfriend of five years still backslides despite her considerable talents as a diplomat, first tried announcing that if she ever caught him drinking again she would leave him. He did drink; then she discovered she loved him too much to carry out her threat. Crying wolf on other occasions had washed away many a line in the sand, and she knew that if this one were to withstand the tide it would have to be deeply etched and skillfully negotiated. First Jenna laid out the problem: "I feel you need to stop drinking, and I also feel that if you can't, our relationship will not last." Next she gave her lover fair warning of the plan she was putting into action: "I am going to be after you about it, checking up on you about it, confronting you about it. I'm sorry if that makes you feel hounded, and I will certainly try to be trusting, but this is a big issue for me. Since you seem to have trouble addressing it on your own, I intend to address it for my sake and for the sake of our relationship." The drinking and lying about it continued, so Jenna moved on to the last stage of her campaign by telling her partner she seriously intended to leave him. When her lover asked if there was anything he could do to prevent that, Jenna replied that he must acknowledge that the drinking was tied to depression and that the help of a psychiatrist was necessary to address both, and added a further condition—he must promise to stick to whatever medication was prescribed. Instead of the usual foot-dragging, her partner called his HMO and three days later started on antidepressants.

Parents and in-laws each in their own way can be impediments to maintaining boundaries: The former tend to urge immediate divorce—"How can you go on living with someone who makes you so unhappy?"—and the latter are prone to defending their errant offspring, who, they insist, "never behaves that way with us." While friends do offer comfort and support, even the most loyal may eventually grow impatient and push for defection. They find it difficult to understand what seems to them pointless self-sacrifice and may grow impatient after repetitive complaints. What none of these good people, and precious few outsiders, understand is that the essential fallout problem is love. If it could be put aside, depression fallout would be a trial but not a trial by fire. "No matter how angry I get, I still tell my wife how much I love her. Even the sound of her voice makes my heart pound. I know the person I fell in love with is still there," writes Jay on behalf of countless posters. "I can't reach her, but somehow I will because I want her back." That is the conundrum at the heart of depression fallout, and the most difficult to face, but it cannot be solved by love alone. Medical and psychotherapeutic help are needed, too. If you and your mate adopt a partnership approach to depression's treatment, the solution will be far easier to find.

# 5

# A Partnership
# Approach to
# Treatment

Writing about depression fallout has cast me in the role of unofficial psychiatric adviser to friends, friends of friends, and even total strangers on planes or in the gym. Everyone seems to have been touched by depression in some manner and wants to talk about a parent, a child, a lover with this illness who has sought or refused treatment. The questions they pose reveal an encouraging increase in the number of people who believe that depression is an illness rather than a state of mind and is treatable with medication and/or psychotherapy, but the information they possess about the specifics of treatment is at best rudimentary and often downright wrong. If I ask what medication a spouse is taking and at what dosage, or what brand of therapy has been sought, or ask for the credentials of the doctor or psychotherapist, my questioners look bewildered, as though such information lay beyond their scope of concern. Yet if the illness at issue were cancer or heart disease, the patient's spouse would be an expert, would talk to the doctors, would search the Internet for information, and would be an active and informed participant at every stage.

The same supportive participation is called for in depression. This chapter covers the essentials of depression pharmacology and psychotherapy, and will enable depressed and non-depressed partners to approach treatment as a cooperative venture. Knowledge is power; choices should be informed by an appreciation of the advantages and limitations of any treatment. Asking the right questions of the professionals reduces uncertainty and stress, and will help both partners assess progress, or lack of it, more accurately. If treatment is left solely to physicians, the likelihood of success is diminished by their often reflexive response: "Here's a prescription for some pills that ought to put you back in form in no time." If the patient then takes sole charge, he or she may take the pills for a week or two and, noting no perceptible change in mood or troubled by side effects, leave the bottle in the medicine cabinet. Persistent depression sufferers will return to the doctor (or consult a new doctor) and receive an alternate antidepressant, but be given no further information other than an assurance that this new one will do the trick; for not a few, this is an empty promise. Others will join the ranks of the half-well; while their depression weighs less heavily, it still makes its presence known. Problems like these do double damage by dashing hopes for improvement and permitting further deterioration of the relationship. Non-depressed partners who avoid involvement in their mates' treatment risk both outcomes.

The depressed are neither good questioners nor listeners. Information skips in one ear and out the other or is mangled by their moods, and they are not the best judges of their progress. If I were Commissioner of Depression, I would insist that a concerned family member or friend read this chapter, sit in on office visits, ask the doctor to repeat instructions, and take notes on what is said. Both the depressed and the fallout partner would be required to independently jot down daily observations, such as "No change at all but slept better" and "Mary (or Dick) much calmer, less argumentative," and compare them once a week. If six weeks passed without significant improvement, despite careful monitoring and following any suggested dosage adjustment, the couple would automatically return to the doctor and ask what the next treatment step will be and why. Fallout partners would take a minicourse in supportive techniques. They would learn how to show interest in treatment without giving the impression that they are attempting to control it, and to encourage Mary or Dick by pointing out that sleeping better is significant, that their irritability quotient is markedly lower, and that they are much more like their old selves again.

Solicitude has its limits. Keeping optimism afloat without undue interference calls for delicacy. It's no fun to be put under a microscope and examined; if you interpret every word or gesture as "evidence" of something good or bad, you will make your partner uncomfortably self-conscious.

Instead, acknowledge improvement with deeds: give more hugs, smile more often, suggest doing more together, and respect the need of the depressed to be alone at times.

Both partners will benefit from the following grounding in the basics of psychopharmacological and psychothera- peutic treatments for depression.

## PHARMACOLOGY 101

The treatment of psychiatric illness has a long and some- times intemperate history. Ancient Greeks suffering from "melancholia" were thought to have an excess of black bile, one of the bodily fluids called "humours," then believed responsible for moods and personality. Hip- pocrates recommended a change of diet and herbal reme- dies to eliminate its excess, a more humane choice than that of the Phoenicians, who piled the depressed into boats and set them adrift on the high seas. Western thought has always been more severe than Eastern in deal- ing with this illness: While we were burning "witches" at the stake, in the East the psychiatrically disturbed were often revered as seers favored by the gods. In nineteenth- century England and well into the twentieth, psychiatrists viewed the mentally ill as aliens, troublemakers, and bio- logical degenerates and promoted eugenics in "the hope that the collective wisdom [of the Medico-Psychological Association of Great Britain] might evolve a practical scheme whereby a polluting stream might be dammed and great good thus accrue to the national health."

In 1867, an English physician addressing the all-male

Obstetrical Society felt it necessary to speak out against removal of the clitoris of "insane" females, a practice then approved by such eminences as the Archbishop of Canterbury and the Princess of Wales. In the early twentieth century, for Virginia Woolf and others of her sex and class, confinement in a private sanatorium and doses of potentially fatal sleeping potions were prescribed while men were considered to be "eccentric."

As recently as the 1960s, during the American heyday of psychoanalysis, mothers of autistic, bipolar, and schizophrenic children were callously blamed for their offsprings' disturbed state of mind, even though the Food and Drug Administration had approved the first antidepressants and antipsychotics, and the benefits of lithium as a therapeutic drug for manic depression were already known. By 1987, when Prozac blazed its way into the headlines, most Americans, including an outsize slice of mental health professionals, considered depression to be solely an illness of the mind, not the brain. Widespread denial of depression by its sufferers is proof that this view still flourishes.

As the gap between neurology and psychiatry closes and scientists probe more precisely into the brain's complexity, today's methods of diagnosing and treating depressive illness will be regarded as crude and imprecise. Instead of conducting a brief interview with patients, followed by a prescription for an antidepressant bestseller, doctors will use blood tests and imaging technology to map the brain's terrain and assess damage to it, and then prescribe a corrective treatment tailored to each individual.

They will be mindful of childhood experiences that may have altered the brain's circuitry and will routinely demand a thorough physical examination—including a close look at thyroid function—to check for evidence of coexisting illnesses that are linked to depression. The range of treatments at their disposal will broaden dramatically when ongoing research translates into approved new treatments, and their efficacy will be accurately measured.

For now, treatment is conducted by trial and error, as though depression sufferers were peas in a pod. If the first drug fails, a second is prescribed; sometimes another is added to address the side effects that antidepressants can provoke. A study of 337 depressed patients enrolled in a health care program revealed that almost one-third of them were subsequently either switched to another medication, put on a higher dose, had a second drug added, or were taken off the drugs due to adverse reactions and unpleasant side effects. While no information is given about the quality of patient-doctor communication in this and similar studies, the National Depressive and Manic-Depressive Association believes that in general it is subpar; in their recent poll of one thousand patients, more than half had stopped taking their medication due to uncomfortable side effects.

But there is much good news to report as well. The currently available antidepressants, which fall into four categories, will, if skillfully used, help between 60 and 70 percent of all depression sufferers, and there are other effective treatments if these fail. Most frequently prescribed are the SSRIs (selective serotonin reuptake inhibitors), which include Prozac, Zoloft, Paxil, Luvox, and Celexa; the first three make up a hefty share of the antidepressants prescribed in this country. All specifically target the neurotransmitter serotonin on the unproven supposition, suggested by animal models, that it is key to mental health and that depression lowers its levels in the brain. But since these drugs immediately affect serotonin levels yet their full effects on depression are not seen for weeks, serotonin appears to initiate a long cascade reaction in the brain. The popularity of the SSRIs rests more with their relative freedom from side effects than with their efficacy. In terms of results, they are no more effective than their predecessors, the tricyclic antidepressants (TCAs): Elavil, Anafranil, Norpramin, Tofranil, and Pamelor; all of these affect serotonin and also norepinephrine, another neurotransmitter implicated in depression. The so-called atypical antidepressants, including Wellbutrin, Serzone, Effexor, and Asendin, differ structurally and operate on multiple neurotransmitter systems. Wellbutrin has the added advantage of suppressing the desire to smoke and is marketed for that purpose under the brand name Zyban.

Atypical depression, which confusingly has nothing to do with atypical antidepressants, afflicts up to 40 percent of all depression sufferers, but even psychiatrists very often miss the diagnosis. While an SSRI may provide partial and temporary relief, atypical depression responds best to the fourth category of drugs, the MAOIs (monoamine oxidase inhibitors). These medications inhibit the breakdown of serotonin, norepinephrine, and a third neurotransmitter, dopamine. The MAOIs available in this country—Nardil,

Morplan, and Parnate—have one serious drawback: a potentially fatal reaction to many foods and beverages (among them cold cuts and cured meats, most fermented cheeses, overripe bananas, and Chianti), and also to some popular over-the-counter drugs. If these are carelessly ingested, a telltale pounding, back-of-the-head headache and racing pulse ensue, signaling a precipitous spike in blood pressure. While users can take a blocker pill that stops this reaction cold, MAOIs are underprescribed despite their efficacy. Having had such a reaction in a Paris bistro while eating boeuf bourguignon, and subsequently discovering pinhead bits of sausage in it, I can attest to the sheer terror of knowing that nothing stood between me and mortality except an enormous white pill that looked like something a veterinarian might prescribe for a rhinoceros.

Sufferers of atypical depression can now eat and drink with abandon and enjoy sex, thanks to RIMAs (reversible monoamine inhibitors). Although used extensively in Europe and elsewhere, RIMAs are not yet available in the United States because their manufacturer, hoping for a larger share of the market, chose to conduct the necessary Food and Drug Administration trials as a medication for social phobia rather than for depression, a grievous miscalculation on their part. Knowledgeable psychopharmacologists can send an RIMA prescription to a pharmacy in Canada that will deliver them to you by mail. Any physician willing to go the extra mile on behalf of atypical patients can fill out a form and receive from the FDA a so-called Compassionate IND number that allows the package to pass through U.S. Customs without problems, providing not more than six hundred pills are ordered at one time. For the overlooked sufferers of atypical depression, the benefits of RIMAs more than compensate for the lack of health insurance reimbursement.

It is an uncomfortable truth that the doctor's choice of medication is influenced by intensive marketing on the part of pharmaceutical companies. The marketing goal is to induce brand loyalty. Sales agents, competing for a share in the multibillion-dollar antidepressant market, dispense free samples of drugs and gifts—pens, coffee cups, golf balls, anything that can be emblazoned with a logo—and pay doctors to attend dinners where an "expert" will extol the benefits of their particular product. All of the products have undergone the clinical and efficacy (but not maintenance) trials required by the FDA, but the costly trials are financed and conducted by the drug's manufacturer, who has likely paid participating doctors a "per head" fee for each patient recruited. The product ads that now turn up regularly in newspapers, magazines, and on television promote name recognition among patients; when handed a prescription for Prozac, Zoloft, or Paxil, they feel comfortable and assume that wellness is on the way.

As already noted, wellness often needs a lot of coaxing. One patient may do well on an SSRI drug that makes another edgy and sleepless, while a third user may oversleep, feel nauseous, or have headaches. Often, a switch of brand or of drug classification will work, as will adding a second drug to the mix. Even though RIMAs are the basis for my well-being, like many other depression sufferers I also take an antidepressant called trazadone to help me sleep. It is not all that unusual for someone whose depression is severe to take three or four drugs, particularly if anxiety is an additional problem. Lurking on the sidelines are the sexual effects discussed in Chapter 7; combating them may call for yet more pills. Knowing that one is dependent on an array of tablets and capsules, for all the relief they bring, is unsettling. Many users worry that they will forget to pack them for a trip, or that their wise psychiatrist will retire, or that some catastrophic event will block access to the supply of pharmaceutical agents that keep them going.

Dosage and timing are important, too. The recommended average dose of any given antidepressant does not mean that it is necessarily the right dose for every user, and whatever dose serves for "average" times may prove insufficient during high-stress periods. Sometimes medication takes effect within ten days and relief comes with the startling rapidity of a shade snapping up, but change is usually more gradual and may require up to twelve weeks at the optimal dose. If the medication has not produced any results within this time frame, an alternative medication should be tried, but changing drugs from one day to the next can be a problem. Patients on SSRIs must remain drug-free for a fortnight—and for five weeks if they have been taking Prozac, which takes a long time to clear out of the system—before starting on an MAOI or an RIMA, and going off Paxil appears to create such severe problems for some users that a class-action suit has been brought against its manufacturer. When the change in mood is incremental or incomplete, depression sufferers, inclined to negative thinking, often assume that nothing good has happened despite their partners' observations to the contrary. When patients lose sight of the tradeoff between their pre- and post-medication states, they may start skipping pills or discontinue them. Each time this happens, the illness is more difficult to dislodge.

Just short of half of all depression sufferers who seek professional help receive it from primary care physicians, not specialists. Given the time constraints imposed on HMO doctors and the complex nature of this illness, it is not surprising that patients are poorly informed about the treatments offered. Those who go directly to a psychiatrist, or are referred to one, are more likely to receive individualized treatment to the extent that today's science permits, but knowing the right questions to ask can make a big difference in outcome. Psychopharmacologists, many of whom are respected researchers in their own right, are less likely to be found on HMO rosters. They are expensive, charging fees as high as $600 for an initial visit, but they often succeed where others have failed. These experts are usually to be found in hospitals with excellent psychiatric departments and can be seen on a consultation basis. Their reputations help ensure that the prescribing doctor will accept (although sometimes grudgingly) and correctly implement their advice. Patients should provide them with a history of treatment to date—what drugs for how long at what dosage, side effects, and improvements noted—so as to avoid retracing steps already taken.

Those who are not helped by medication will eventually be advised to try electroconvulsive treatment (ECT), and at least half of them will get their life back as a result. The prospect is undeniably daunting, but the reality is otherwise and bears no resemblance to the outmoded methods that once earned ECT a bad name. Patients are given a short-acting anesthetic that puts them out for fifteen minutes, and the actual shock administered—the electrical equivalent of the output of a hundred-watt bulb—lasts only one second. On waking up, there may be short-term memory loss. ECT takes effect sooner than medication, and most ECT patients' depression improves substantially within a few weeks of treatment. The usual practice is to give ten to twelve treatments over six weeks, often on an outpatient basis. Booster treatments may be recommended, just as continuing drug therapy is necessary for pill takers, but many ECT patients are still free of depression a full year after treatment.

A hospital is the safest place for a severely depressed patient who is at risk of suicide or has become psychotic. Round-the-clock supervision assures that medications will be taken until the worst has passed, and doctors are on hand if anything untoward happens. Patients and families can disabuse themselves of outmoded tales of involuntary incarceration that stretches into weeks or months. The dictates of their bottom line ensure that HMOs will be as eager as the hospitals to discharge their patients within a few days; complaints are more often of involuntary release. The principal problems will be that no one has time to answer questions and that patients are released before it can be determined if the drug used is really helpful.

Participation in treatment extends beyond knowing

what medication(s) a depressed partner is taking. Good communication between the physician and the non-depressed mate is as important as between physician and patient. Experienced doctors will welcome some input from a close observer of their patient's behavior on home territory. The mere act of sitting in a doctor's office spurs the depressed to minimize the extent to which their depression cripples them. They often raise themselves, Lazarus-like, from a near-catatonic state and chattily inform the physician that maybe they've been feeling a bit under the weather lately, but it's nothing they can't handle. Side effect complaints go unmentioned, whereas at home they are pronounced intolerable and positive effects are overlooked. This is, again, the Dr. Jekyll defense mechanism at work.

Even the gutsiest of depression sufferers contemplate suicide. They will rarely admit this to a doctor, even when directly questioned, but according to Message Board partners, threats of suicide are quite common during emotional scenes. Non-depressed mates, accustomed to melodrama, complain that threatening suicide is often used by their partners as a poor-me, attention-getting ploy, but non-depressed people don't think about killing themselves. Some threats may be melodramatic manipulation while others will be real, and it is hard to tell the difference.

The National Depressive and Manic-Depressive Association has a list of specific recommendations for family members and friends who believe someone they know is at risk of committing suicide, the first of which is to take suicidal ideation and threats, and attempts seriously. Stay calm, but don't underreact; express concern, listen attentively, maintain eye contact, and, if appropriate, use reassuring body language, such as moving closer and holding your mate's hand. Acknowledge his or her feelings; be empathetic, not judgmental. Most important of all, call the prescribing physician and/or therapist even if your partner says this is not necessary; alternatively, contact a crisis intervention service or call 911.

## Herbal and Other Remedies for Depression

Depression has been around for five millennia or more, and the use of plants and roots to alleviate it has a long history. Taking a so-called natural substance sounds benign to uninformed ears, but just because something grows wild in the fields does not mean that it is necessarily good for you—witness marijuana and poisonous mushrooms. The costly and time-consuming safety and efficacy trials required by the Food and Drug Administration for prescription drugs do not apply to such over-the-counter products as St. John's wort, ginkgo biloba, valerian, kava, and SAM-e, among others, and their manufacturers are free to make unsubstantiated claims. While a number of studies—many of them poorly designed—have been conducted on the efficacy of herbal substances for depression, research has been hampered by the chemical complexity of the products and the lack of standardization of commonly available preparations. A further drawback is that their effectiveness has been measured only in comparison to a placebo, not to a prescription antidepressant. The National Institutes of Health has undertaken a major study of herbal versus prescription drugs, but the results will not be in for some time.

As St. John's wort gained a reputation for mitigating the symptoms of mild to moderate depression in Germany, where standardization is subject to more control than it is here, sales in the United States began to billow, and enough users reported improvement to cause a stir in the popular press. The media have been less attentive to its side effects, news of which is accumulating: St. John's wort can decrease the effectiveness of oral contraceptives, cholesterol-lowering drugs, calcium-channel blockers for high blood pressure and coronary heart disease, and protease inhibitors for HIV infection. When I asked my psychopharmacologist if I could lower my RIMA dose by supplementing it with some St. John's wort, he explained that since both affect monoamine oxidase, the combination could be dangerous, yet mention of this contraindication is rare even in the professional literature.

The lack of controls on herbal remedies renders dosage problematic, as a journalist at the *Los Angeles Times* discovered. When samples of ten different brands of St. John's wort were sent to an independent laboratory for analysis, the amount of hypericin (the component used for standardization purposes) varied from 20 to 140 percent of the amount claimed on the label, with half the brands containing less than 80 percent of the labeled amount.

A nonprescription supplement called SAM-e made

headlines in 1999 and has been reported as helpful, but certainly less so than the grandiose claims made in its behalf. A full-page *New York Times* advertisement for a book about SAM-e described it as "a supplement that can conquer depression safely and naturally in a matter of days." Although some European trials have compared SAM-e to imipramine, a TCA, and found the two to be equal in their effectiveness for depression, the book's author, a psychiatrist, uses SAM-e primarily as an adjunct to the antidepressant medications he prescribes for his patients.

As the above indicates, wandering into a health-products store and picking from among the multiple offerings is not the best way to deal with depression, nor is it risk-free. Research indicates that a program of regular aerobic exercise can beat their record, even when the depression is severe.

## A Situation Report from the Message Board

Going on an antidepressant produces changes in behavior that do not always register in the minds of users, inviting the possibility of discouragement and discontinuation of medication. Fallout partners who are good observers and supporters can prevent this from happening. Layla had reported to the Message Board that her husband and she had been disappointed with his limited response to Wellbutrin, but when Serzone was added several months later she noted changes that spoke volumes about his improved biochemistry. Her husband had cut down on his drinking, begun spontaneously giving her little hugs and kisses, and now told her he loved her and wanted to be more affectionate, all without his previous tone of sad desperation. Out golfing with her one weekend, he broke into song when it rained and danced a jig on the green. When arguments erupted, her husband sprang back to normal after a couple of hours instead of brooding for days, and he was relaxed and talkative around their friends. His professional life took an upturn as well; he began working on a new project, had more lunches with his coworkers, and even came home one day after a conversation about desserts and asked Layla for her cookie recipe so he could whip up a batch to share with them.

Layla's husband was far less aware of all these changes than she. While he told her he was sleeping better and dreaming more, and noticed on a few occasions that he was a bit more outgoing than usual, for the most part he seemed to think that not much had changed. "I find this interesting not only because he seems very different to me," she wrote, "but also because he made the same statements about the Wellbutrin and wanted to stop taking it because he thought it had no effect on him." To her surprise, the improvements in her husband's mood made Layla feel off-kilter. "I think what's happening is that he's being way more pleasant and personable, but that hasn't really made life 'all better.'" Some part of her, she said, had expected clear sailing if they could just reach this kind of breakthrough, but her husband still didn't pay the bills on time, hadn't started psychotherapy as promised, and wasn't taking any of the daily living responsibilities off her shoulders. "I don't want to feel this way," she declared.

"I want to feel energized and encouraged and hopeful, and, darn it, I deserve to because I've worked very hard to get us to this point. And I worry horribly that the pills may stop working in the future and we'll be back at square one again. Any suggestions?"

I give gold stars to Layla for all her hard work—it has paid off handsomely. If for some unforeseen reason the medications do stop working, the prospects for further solutions are enhanced by the fact that the prescribing psychiatrist appears to be knowledgeable and inventive. In what will probably be a very long meantime, she should enjoy and demonstrably respond to her partner's pleasant and personable demeanor; find ways to let him know how differently he acts now with her and with others; suggest to him that he write down a sentence or two every day summing up how he feels so that the changes will be more evident to him; and ask if he would like to start with a joint therapy session ("It's our relationship so it's our problem"). And Layla could perhaps tell her husband that she will take over paying the bills for the next few months.

The depressive population seems to be divided into those sufferers who see their meds as life's blood and those who can't wait to stop taking them. Every report on a depressed partner who has fallen off the antidepressant wagon is met with a collective groan. If persuading your partner to go on antidepressants was a titanic struggle, be prepared for a blithe announcement at some point that they are no longer necessary. Don't believe it. Doctors recommend continuing medication—called "maintenance treatment"—for a minimum of six months after their optimal effects kick in, but that would be poor advice for someone on their third, or even second episode of depression; further, a supposed first bout may have been preceded by others not recognized as such. As already noted, depressions wax and wane, so it is feasible that, in some cases, stopping the pills would not have an immediately noticeable impact on mood, but when the illness gathers force again, the descent will be rapid and more resistant to treatment than before.

The prudent answer to maintenance treatment is to put it firmly in the hands of the medicating psychiatrist; no one else is a good judge of the right course to follow. Even when there are no apparent problems, quarterly visits to the doctor (usually required for refills of prescriptions) are the only secure way to keep on top of the illness. The need to adjust dosages is not unusual; the optimal dose for a prolonged period may at another time cause agitation and interfere with sleep, while during particularly stressful times a higher dose may be needed. One last piece of information to share with your partner: Antidepressants should be stopped gradually, not abruptly. Going cold turkey can cause a lot of problems.

## PSYCHOTHERAPY 101

In the fifteen years since my depression was first diagnosed I have done a gradual 180-degree turn vis-à-vis the benefits of psychotherapy and now count myself among its advocates. Medication saved my life, but with the concurrent aid of a first-class psychotherapist I would have come far sooner to the insights I now possess about the interpersonal ramifications of my depression and the self-defeating thoughts and behavior that are its chosen companions.

My first face-to-face experience with a therapist is worth relating because it shows that therapy for depression works best when the therapist is familiar with the illness and its mindset, and is not ruled by the Freudian teaching that still dominates graduate schools of psychology and social work. The problem I handed to my therapist was a long and dismal record of conflict-ridden relationships, and general feelings of malaise and discontent—the self-diagnosis of many undiagnosed depressives. Although she claimed expertise in the faster-acting, problem-solving therapeutic approaches then coming into vogue, my therapist decided early on that all my problems derived from the disappearance of my father when I was only an infant. She had little interest in discussing my mother's influence over my feelings and behavior, nor did she ever address my symptoms of depression and their need for medical attention. Despite the promise to help me tackle current problems, we talked only of the past, and I was instructed to paste my father's face on each male countenance in my dreams. In eighteen months I had made little progress under her tutelage, and my depression galloped on.

Only recently did I discover for myself how effective good psychotherapy can be for a depression sufferer. When some bad news started a downward spiral, I tried all my usual tricks to steer clear of the abyss, but with each passing day my despair deepened. Then came a lifeline: the name of a psychotherapist who had helped a severely depressed friend. I was so awash in insights after three sessions that I had to take a month off to absorb them before going back two more times. This therapist knew about atypical depression and so could help me assess my reactions to what had happened in the light of its symptoms; he was a good listener and made specific suggestions about how I could deal with my distress. At the end of the fifth session, I felt I was once again in control of my emotions and could cope with the situation alone, and the psychotherapist, instead of insisting that I keep coming, assured me that should the need arise, he would be there to help me again.

This recent therapy experience speaks to the limits of medication: First, the barrier it erects against depression may crumble in the face of stress, and second, it cannot work behavioral miracles. A negative mode of thinking, like any bad habit, is easy to acquire and difficult to break. In as short a time as six months, depression's bleak outlook on the self and the world becomes ingrained. While antidepressants bring back the will to change, the *how* and *what* to change is a formidable challenge to meet on one's own. Having a therapist is like having a coach who knows the rules and tricks of the game and can point out mistakes, exhorting you to do your best and applauding progress.

Before medication came along, psychotherapy was the only alternative to waiting out the depression or living with it permanently. The elites of psychotherapy were the psychoanalysts, whose goal was a virtual restructuring of one's personality—a feat that allegedly required up to five hours a week on the couch for years and years, and very little input from the analyst other than an occasional "And how do you feel about that?" Analysts, Freudian to the core, did not believe in medication and, in the opinion of one psychiatrist, often mistook their patients for an annuity. With the advent of Prozac and cost-minded HMOs, two forms of short-term therapy gained credence: cognitive-behavioral therapy (CBT) and interpersonal therapy (IPT).

Both CBT and IPT focus on the present rather than the past and are designed to help patients see what they are doing wrong and alter their way of thinking and behaving. For those who are subject to defeatist thoughts about themselves and the world, who automatically expect everything to turn out for the worst and who rate themselves as ineffective and inadequate, cognitive-behavioral therapy (CBT) is a good choice. If the problem is constant embroilment in conflicts with friends and coworkers, and if love affairs always turn sour, interpersonal therapy (IPT), designed specifically as a treatment for depression, may be more suitable. These and other short-term therapies share certain rules. They are usually time-limited (eight to sixteen weekly sessions); their emphasis is on changing current behavior and thinking; they require self-monitoring of change and progress and often involve "homework" between sessions; and the therapist is active and directive.

Choosing a therapist who will work well for you is part luck, part preliminary groundwork. Start by canvassing your friends for recommendations and then ask some questions of the therapist before making an appointment: Do you have experience in working with depression sufferers or with their partners? Stay clear of those who say no.

Do you practice one of the short-term therapies designed to address a specific problem, or do you work on an open-ended basis? The former will be more helpful to most fall-out partners than the latter. Do you hold a degree in psychology and how long have you been in practice? Solid credentials and experience are in your favor. What is your attitude toward antidepressant medication, and do you have a referral list of doctors if you believe it is indicated? A positive response to both is important.

Note the manner in which the answers are given. If the therapist seems reluctant to respond, as though you were imposing on his or her time, of if they propose a date far into the future, go on to the next name on your list. If after a couple of sessions the patient-therapist fit seems poor, cut things short and try someone else. Not much will be accomplished if the relationship isn't a good one, and continuing will eat into the number of sessions your HMO will cover.

## Some Psychotherapy Caveats

Attempts to justify a particular type of talk therapy as the best one for depression ring hollow because different people have wildly varying psyches and lives. Research studies that have assembled small groups of depressed people, treated half with CBT and half with IPT, and then proclaimed one therapy to be superior are inconclusive. Some people start off with useful insights and need only be made aware that their repetitive behavioral patterns are closely tied to their depression, and others need many sessions before even accepting a diagnosis of depression. A recently widowed spouse who has become depressed needs one kind of help, while a long-depressed partner needs another. Many depressed people have both interpersonal problems and a negative view of themselves and the world around them. In the view of one psychiatrist, the more "cognitive" the problem, the more unsuccessful the therapy may be since it forces the patient to confront what he or she cannot change. What count most in successful psychotherapy are the skills, insights, and experience of the therapist who provides it.

Established psychotherapists are trained and receive a license awarding them the title of psychologist, but anyone can claim to be a therapist and hang out a shingle that says THERAPY AVAILABLE HERE. According to the *Harvard Mental Health Letter,* there are no less than four hundred varieties of therapy on offer, hardly any of which have been tested for results. Unless you are willing to be a guinea pig, the safest course is to pick a practitioner with a good reputation, but this does not guarantee good results. Liking and trusting one's therapist is all-important. I liked my first therapist when I started, but that soon changed. New to the ways of therapy, I made a typical mistake in assuming that she knew best, and that I was manifesting yet more signs of interpersonal deficits. Moreover, there was the exit problem: I didn't want to hurt her feelings; had invested effort, time, and money in her services; was afraid I couldn't find somebody else. Another lesson: Worry about your feelings, not your therapist's, and ask your friends for the name of someone who has helped them.

Any psychotherapist who rejects medication out of hand should be prohibited from accepting patients who are or may be depressed. The either-or turf battle that once raged fiercely is yesterday's news and most talk therapists and prescription-writing psychiatrists now agree that the two approaches work best in tandem, but there are still many holdouts from the traditional school of psychology. A psychotherapist who hems and haws when asked for an opinion on antidepressants and has no referral list of psychiatrists is waving a red flag.

The best therapists are willing to adapt to their patients' needs and do what's best for the individual. One practitioner, when asked what qualities he would look for in a psychotherapist said, "A lively intelligence and compassion, an open mind free of dogma, a track record on depression, and a manner that put me immediately at ease, and while I would expect him or her to be a good listener, I would also expect a lot of feedback."

## Inside a Therapist's Office

Neal Aponte, a clinical psychologist who resists being labeled but says his approach could be described as psychodynamic, meets all the above criteria, and his practice includes both depression and depression fallout sufferers.

The value of treating many patients with a common problem is that shared patterns of thinking and feeling emerge. The depressed and their partners believe they are in virgin territory, but their respective journeys follow well-trodden paths. Aponte's depressed patients, for example, consistently use the same graphic images when talking about their depression: a cosmic black hole whose force they can't resist; a whirlpool of strange, morbid feelings and thoughts that sucks them down into its eddy; a powerful internal beast with which they are wrestling in the dark. Depressed patients feel that they are up against something much larger than themselves, "as though a force over which they have no control and cannot escape had taken control of them," he explains. "For them, the deterioration of the relationship serves to reinforce the despair and the harsh, bleak outlook typical of this illness. He, or she, sees himself as lacking—stupid, incompetent, clumsy, unlovable, lazy, ugly, and a host of other negatives. Because he views the world around him in the same way he experiences his internal world, the patient applies the same hypercritical judgments to his partner that he applies to himself."

Dr. Aponte's fallout patients consistently describe their depressed mates as being in hiding or locked away out of reach somewhere, or of having been taken over by someone else. They don't know where their original partner has gone and can't any longer make emotional or physical contact with him or her. "Unable to recognize the person they were attracted to and fell in love with, they're in mourning for the relationship as they once knew it. The anguish they convey—their sense of loss, sorrow, and frustration—comes across very powerfully, as does the loneliness and feelings of abandonment that this loss engenders." Both partners, Aponte points out, are actually talking about the same thing; both "have the sense that the relationship has been hijacked by the depression. Combine these two perspectives—one from the inside, the other from the outside looking in—and you have a "combustible situation just waiting to explode."

A repeated complaint of non-depressed partners is that they are forced into a caretaking role. One can be the most compassionate, understanding, loving man or woman in the world, "but it's next to impossible to live with someone who is sour, bitter, frequently angry, constantly complaining, and who is increasingly withdrawn and socially isolated," says Aponte. "That's going to generate a lot of charged feelings—resentment, frustration, anger, even hate, and often guilt as well for not being compassionate enough."

Queried about depression's seeming ability to erase the good memories shared together, Aponte explained that although a memory file remains, sufferers see their life prior to the depressive episode as though it were someone else's. They find it difficult to relate those memories to their current life, he says, and may express such thoughts as "Given who I am now, how was I ever able to attract such a wonderful person? What did she (or he) see in me in the first place?" While Aponte does see a number of depressives who become hostile and critical of partners, "projecting what they feel internally onto the world around them," in his clinical experience the former view predominates.

One is left to wonder why, given so much inner self-criticism, the depressed aren't able to change their ways. Aponte's view is that "for all of us, depressed or not, the hardest things to acknowledge and face up to are the things we know in our hearts to be true. Much of human behavior is irrational and illogical, so just having insight usually isn't enough," he says, which is where the mental health professional comes in. "I haven't any set formula. There are always signposts and a road map, but the actual journey will be determined by patient and therapist together."

That journey includes helping the patient to acknowledge the presence of depression. Dr. Aponte can't remember a case where a depressed person was able to completely mask his depression because "it oozes out of their pores. You can't hide it because in a sense it's who you are." There's often a big reservoir of shame and guilt about being depressed, and this has to be respected and worked with, not shoved aside. The societal stigma reinforces self-defeatism and plays into the depressed person's sense of being unworthy of love, of being inadequate and somehow less than human. "A patient may say to me, 'Why do I need to come to a damn therapist? If I were tough enough I'd be able to manage this on my own, just like my mother did.' Of course, Mother may have drunk herself into oblivion or watched television all day, and never had a job. It's important to help patients see how their illness is compromising their lives."

Sooner or later Dr. Aponte will point out to his depressed patients how exhausting it is to keep up a front when they're falling apart inside, and will suggest getting a medical opinion on the patient's depression. "Nine times out of ten, it's a relief to them to be able to put a name to their problem, but going on meds, altering their brain chemistry, scares a lot of people. I tell them that a consultation doesn't necessarily commit them to taking antidepressants, but it's part of my job to dispel misinformation about them. Psychotherapy plus medication is the optimal treatment."

## Some Advice for Fallout Partners

Looking through this keyhole into a good therapist's office underscores the value of suggesting psychotherapy to mates who refuse to see a doctor; the unbiased opinion and advice of a professional stand a better chance of acceptance than the views of a spouse or lover. But psychotherapy is a profoundly personal affair, and most who enter it are reluctant to discuss what's going on unless they are extremely enthusiastic about how it is progressing. Rule number one for non-depressed partners is to restrain from meddling in the process, even when the perceived results are not to their liking. When a patient reports that the therapist agrees he or she is probably in a bad relationship, and that they are not depressed, the temptation to jeer and boo is hard to resist. Hassling over who is right is useless; if the bond between therapist and patient has been made, criticizing the therapist will only serve to strengthen it. Bear in mind, however, that the message conveyed is not always an accurate rendition of what the therapist said. Further, as Dr. Aponte makes clear, psychotherapy doesn't adhere to a strict timetable, and the track to self-understanding is subject to detours.

A prevalent complaint of fallout partners is that they have no opportunity to present their side of the problem to the therapist. When Lila's husband, during his second year of therapy, came home with the news that he had reported her side of the story to his therapist and been told on the spot that he was controlling and manipulative and was forcing his wants and needs on others with predictable results, Lila asked the Message Board why this hadn't happened long ago. It seemed to her that if the therapist was supposed to be helping her husband, she should have been invited to come for a joint session early in the process. The post elicited similar complaints from others. A fallout husband said that when his wife asked the therapist if he could come with her to a session, the therapist replied that he hadn't "finished with my wife yet, and that when he wanted to see me he would let me know."

Psychotherapists field the question of partner exclusion by emphasizing the importance to the patient of feeling safe and point out that confidentiality, the first commandment of therapists, is the only way to ensure it; the sole exception all therapists are willing to make is when a patient is a suicide risk or a danger to others. If I were to put on my depressed hat, I would wholeheartedly agree, but were I wearing my fallout hat, I would lobby hard to be included. The Happy Couple facade isn't easy to penetrate, and many depressed mates fool their therapists into thinking that the only product of their depression is personal sorrow made more intense by an unsympathetic partner. This may well have been what transpired during the initial eighteen months of Lila's husband's therapy; if asked for an explanation, the therapist might have said that the patient had not been "ready" to address the issue and that forcing him to face it prematurely would solve nothing.

The logic of involving the partner is in my view irrefutable, and some therapists do agree that a joint session from time to time is helpful. No matter what the therapist's view on this issue, he or she won't welcome telephone calls from non-depressed partners reporting the latest wrinkle in their patients' demeanor at home. The best way to gain entry into the process is to persuade your depressed mate that if you are allowed to sit in on a session from time to time, it will help you to see both sides of the problem, not just your own.

## SUPPORT GROUPS

Mental health organizations run support groups for sufferers of unipolar and bipolar depression, and also for their friends and family. When I inquired about attending the friends and family group run by the Mood Disorders Support Group in New York City, I was put by mistake in a support group for depression sufferers. I was in good spirits at the time, but at the end of an evening spent with people so drained by their illness, I could hardly sit upright. Three weeks later, in the right group at last, I discovered that a well-run friends and family group can be an emotional godsend and a source of invaluable advice; if there is such a group within striking distance of your home, take advantage of it. The group's facilitator had taken a mandatory course in the treatment of depressive illness and was a walking encyclopedia. His skill and compassion made every weekly session a lesson in how to cope with fallout, and soon transformed me from observer into active participant.

However, attendees at depression groups may, if their depression is mild, react as I did to three hours in the company of people far worse off and complain that they don't want to sit around with a bunch of "deadbeats" who speak in a monotone. But they will also see firsthand how devastating the illness can be, which in turn can translate into a determination to control their own. The more severely afflicted will feel a sense of solidarity that is invaluable in dispelling the guilt and social isolation that depression fosters. A support group is also a repository of information about old and new medications, side effects, good and bad doctors, insurance, and coping skills. Members know the importance of complying with treatment and are better at policing backsliders than are family members. The most likely to backslide are the bipolar sufferers, whose illness alternates between heady ups and dismal downs and is difficult to control.

## Living Side by Side with a Mercurial Mind

A bipolar support group always includes men and women who are tipping into the early stages of mania; they are the irrepressible chatterboxes and foot jigglers who leap from topic to topic without heed to other participants or the facilitator and are impervious to warnings of impending mania. Their peers who have left mania behind through medication lecture them sternly but are probably envious of the exhilaration on display; in the friends and family group, their partners talk about their preposterous behavior. As you will learn, the best and perhaps only way to live with a bipolar is to establish a partnership approach to treatment that is as foolproof as one can make it. The alternative is to allow your heart to break, and break again.

Howard Smith, facilitator of the friends and family support group I attended, is bipolar; he has tried every new drug and psychotherapeutic treatment (and stuck to them faithfully), but each day is an exercise in determination and hope. Once a well-known journalist, his second career has been devoted to building one of the finest mental health consumer chapters in the country. Howard's life now is very different from the one he led in the days when he hung out with the Beatles and won an Oscar for his documentary on evangelist preachers, but it is both satisfying and productive. The advice that follows is informed by his insights.

For sufferers of manic depression, the driving force behind some of history's most lauded creative artists, most dazzling entrepreneurs, and wiliest of con men, the middle way is hard to find. Though blessed with gifts, manic depressives lack judgment and foresight. Oblivious to stop signs, they go after what they want without thought to consequences—spend money they haven't got (including yours), sleep with whomever they want, and chuck good jobs—not because they are bad people, just because they feel that everything's going to work out okay. Though miserable and contrite when mania is exchanged for depression, bipolars will do it all over again as soon as their spirits start to soar. This wild ride will be repeated up to four times a year, even more often for those who are "rapid cyclers," unless medication intervenes.

In its early upward phase, the manic depressive's charm and optimism are infectious, as a number of Board posters have discovered. The novelistic story of one poster—he chose the screen name Marco Polo—about his whirlwind romance with a fascinating, seductive bipolar woman who broke his heart drew hundreds of responses. Marco Polo's is not a unique tale. If my paternal grandmother were alive today, she would be diagnosed as bipolar. Judged uncontrollable and a probable source of embarrassment to the family, she was turned over to the family lawyer at age eighteen, given a large sum of money, and ensconced in a town one hundred miles away. A famous beauty of her day, and an incorrigible flirt, she zipped through seven husbands and numerous lovers. During summer visits to her home during a brief husbandless period, I was summoned every Sunday morning to read the comics in her gold lamé canopied bed; sometimes I was given hugs and chocolates, at others cruelly berated for being fat and clumsy. By the time my grandmother died, a virtual recluse and with no money, she was as famous for her shocking and imperious behavior as for her multiple marriages.

As the foregoing suggests, dealing with a bipolar partner takes a firm hand and a lot of love. Faith's husband has had the illness for twenty-two of the almost thirty years they have been married; the system designed by Faith, her husband, Jack, and their son protects all three from the worst effects of Jack's illness, and is now a recommended staple in the friends and family group. What makes the system close to foolproof is that Jack's psychiatrist and psychotherapist are part of the team. When her husband starts buying cartons of books on marine biology and decides to shift careers, Faith knows that it's time to call his doctors if he won't do it. One or the other of them will give Jack a ring to ask how he is doing, sparing Faith the need for constant nagging.

Part of Faith's strategy is to claim that her migraine headaches have returned because she knows that her husband's concern for her pain seems to check the progression of his mania just long enough for Jack to become aware of its return. During the downs, Faith and their son, Peter, use humor and their own energy to stir Jack's. The family cat wakes Jack up in the morning, and it is Jack's responsibility to get out of bed and feed him. During the day, all the blinds are up, the windows open, and his favorite music blasts away; Monty Python videos are part of the treatment. Faith tells the support group that their family life was not always so well organized. Years before, when she was overwhelmed and felt close to the edge, she had told her husband that she needed space and was going away for a few months. Jack's first reaction—an angry "Go ahead!"—gave way a few days later to a phone call, pleading that she not leave him alone.

The terms of Faith's return dictated the team approach. The two professional members of the team take her phone calls on nights and weekends if necessary, and they are as familiar with the daily course of Jack's illness as is the family; in their turn, Faith and Peter know as much about Jack's medications as his doctors do. The drugs used to control bipolar illness—lithium, Tegretol, Depakote, and Lamictal, among others—are the heavy guns of the psychopharmacological armamentarium, and they have serious side effects; an antidepressant and an antipsychotic medication are often part of the mix. Trading in the pleasure of exuberant rising mania for a daily drug regime is a constant temptation, and fallout partners must make compliance with treatment the quintessential boundary.

Full partnership in treatment goes beyond unrestricted access to the prescribing doctor and to the psychotherapist. Open, honest communication between partners is always important, but when the illness is manic depression it becomes mandatory. Bipolars do not recognize their symptoms of impending mania, so the well mate must function as an early warning system; incessant talking, no sleep, and grandiose plans signal its arrival. Money—chasing it, spending it, losing it—is a running mania thread, and fallout partners who relinquish responsibility for the family finances may find themselves in bankruptcy. Checking and savings accounts should be in their hands, and their partners should not have credit cards. Non-depressed partners who are cognizant of these dangers, and who insist on the Faith-Jack solution, will help their bipolar beloveds find the middle way. They and their mates can expect a bumpy ride, but it will never be a boring one.

# 6

# The Virtues of
# Being Selfish

Loving someone with a depressive illness puts you on the fast track for loss of self-esteem, a mea culpa approach to the failing relationship, and the conviction that your problem has far more muscle than you do. Getting off that track is difficult because your depressed partner has in a sense become your coach, urging you on to demoralization, the killer third stage of depression fallout. Demoralization is perilously akin to depression, and, for the vulnerable, can open the door wide to the illness itself. But even if your neurotransmitters are up to the job of staving off a true depressive episode, one that might cause your doctor to write a prescription for an antidepressant, you will be hard-pressed to recognize the difference between the real thing and the dreaded stage three. A prolonged stay there is dangerous. Although demoralization cannot be entirely avoided, focusing on your own needs rather than your partner's is a curative strategy that will stave off stress as well.

The dictionary defines the verb *demoralize* as "to deprive a person of spirit, courage, and discipline; to destroy their morale; and to throw them into disorder or confusion." Since nobody sets out to deliberately sabotage his or her own spirit and courage, it follows that if you are demoralized, someone else has initiated the process. In your case, the someone is your depressed mate, but that conclusion isn't always obvious to fallout sufferers for two reasons. The first is that earlier fallout stages have primed you so well for self-doubt and lack of confidence that the constant barrage of criticism and belittlement emanating from your partner drowns out your rational inner voice. Even though you know full well that what is being said is inaccurate and the way you are being treated is unfair, your ability to stand up for yourself and to resist the negativity around you is diminished. The more powerless and hopeless you feel, the more demoralized you will become. The battered relationship will take control and become the focal point of your daily existence.

The second reason is that demoralization has a willful force of its own; given an inch, it burrows a mile down into your psyche and can affect your biology as well. Mimicking depression, demoralization often takes aim at sleeping and eating habits, disturbs concentration and memory, and leaves you with a generalized feeling of physical malaise, as though your body were following the same disturbed course as your mind. One Board poster identifies the deficits of demoralization and ties them up neatly. "I am overwhelmed with worry and hurt and confusion, to the point where I am unable to work, unable to sleep well, eat terribly, don't do anything productive, or much of anything at all," she writes. "It's not that I don't know it would be good for me to do these things, but when I try, I feel so strongly that they are interfering with my ability to concentrate on my problems that I quit trying, not as a conscious choice, but as a compulsion, an obsession."

Compulsion and obsession are powerful instruments of entrapment, an excellent synonym for the no-win endgame kicked off by a partner's depression. "What really plagues me is the uncertainty," writes Sam, expressing the Kafkaesque helplessness of depression-fallout sufferers. "At the slightest hint of displeasure on my part, my depressed wife loses it and starts railing at me. When I tell her how much I love her, she responds that if I did, I wouldn't treat her this way. *What* way?" he asks. "Seems like everything I do is wrong." "I'm living a life that is entirely centered on my depressed husband and the need not to set him off," echoes Tari. "I walk on eggshells, but they always crack, no matter how carefully I tiptoe. I am so tired of feeling like a loser."

In place of grand drama, fallout victims have the sense of living in a soap opera and slip into the habit of writing the script themselves. They anticipate blame and even though they know it is undeserved, it sticks to them. While depression fosters avoidance of responsibility for failure or wrongheadedness, demoralization welcomes it. The proof is in the details of everyday fallout life. Julia's "I'm not depressed" husband cast a pall over Thanksgiving by skipping the predinner festivities, speaking hardly at all during the meal, and leaving before the pumpkin pie on the pretext of office papers he had to read. Julia invited blame for his thoughtless behavior; she apologized for the guest list; for not having put the children at a separate table; for having failed to provide mince pie, as well as pumpkin. "How can I avoid a replay of this at Christmas?" she asked the Message Board. "Is there any way to discuss this with him in a way that won't just get me a headache?"

An affirmative answer would be comforting, but as fallout veterans know, pleasing a depressed person is close to impossible; the illness won't allow it. A discussion becomes an argument lost. Each failed engagement will leave you feeling more trapped, more frustrated and beaten down, because you and your depressed partner are playing games with different rules. Your rules have been in place for a long time and are governed by the love and joint history you share, but depression installed a whole new set of rules while you weren't looking. Since you can't win if you play by them, and you don't want to opt out of the game, you need to figure out how you can hang in there and stay sane until the depression lifts. To do that you have to put your own wants and needs before your partner's and pursue them with single-minded determination. For as long as you cast yourself as the loser in this game, you will have no control over its outcome.

## GWEN'S PUT-YOURSELF-FIRST REGIME

One of childhood's earliest lessons is that we must be considerate of others and aware of their wants and needs, and not push our own agenda to the forefront. Those who fail to learn this lesson, we are told, risk being labeled as selfish, pushy, and thoughtless. Most of us absorb the lesson so well that when we transgress we feel guilty and accuse ourselves of lacking empathy and understanding. Fallout guilt is subdivided into pre- and post-diagnosis of a mate's depression. In the pre-diagnosis stage, you target yourself as the cause of his or her changed behavior. Once the illness has been branded as such by a professional, you embrace the role of supportive caregiver with the enthusiasm of a Florence Nightingale and put your partner's needs first at whatever cost to your own. Each time resentment and anger rise in the face of your partner's cavalier ingratitude, you smother them with reminders that your beloved has an illness. While depression sufferers are often extraordinarily grateful for your devotion and loyalty in the face of their uncaring demeanor, they are unable to express it in recognizable ways. "It isn't his or her fault," you keep reiterating, "I shouldn't be thinking of myself."

But you should be. In your current situation, giving thought to what you need and want is not only acceptable, it is strongly recommended. The advice that follows is specifically addressed to your mental and physical health; like much good advice, it is easier to agree with than to follow. "How am I supposed to do that?" is among the most-asked questions on the Message Board. If a Nobel Prize were given for a feel-good formula, the recipient would be Gwen, long-term partner of a good man in the grip of depression. Despite going through two years of mutual misery, proof that the formula works is in her recent post: "Today I am not only dating but living with a pretty non-depressed depressive and can describe my life as happy." Here is how she got that way.

What triggered the process of Gwen's recovery was a disgusted look at her self-defeating behavior: the extent to which she was bending her life to be "there" for her partner, Alex; behaving like a doormat for his moods; always doing what he wanted so as not to risk a confrontation, and blaming herself if one came anyway. As was evident from the following entries in her journal, none of it was paying off.

*Wednesday*

Slept late. Was on the phone with Alex from 2 A.M. to 4 A.M. He was drunk and lonely. Tried to reassure him and to discuss our relationship. So exhausted got to office at noon. Should have gone to a meeting but stayed in my cubicle instead in case he E-mailed me. Should have worked late but left at 5 P.M. to meet Alex for dinner date he broke yesterday.

*Thursday*

Meant to go running after work but came straight home in case Alex wants to see me tonight. Don't feel like running anyhow. Sent three E-mails hinting about a movie; no response. Flat-out invited him to movie; no response. Bought Cheetos on way home; too upset to cook. Rented a movie he'd like in case he shows up. Watched movie alone. If he wants to see I'll pretend I didn't.

*Friday*

Overslept. Exhausted from 3 A.M. telephone fight. Didn't get any work done. Alex apologized by E-mail. Asked me out dancing tonight. Am worried about his drinking, but want so badly to have some fun with him that said yes. Stayed out later than I wanted. Spent more money than I wanted. Got drunker than I meant to. Alex ran out of cash; I paid for a bunch of his drinks. Big 4 A.M. fight. Up till dawn trying to repair damage.

### Saturday

Don't know how long Alex is staying; don't want to miss a chance to make up so didn't mow lawn. Wanted to watch something on TV, but he had remote. Don't want to drive him away by asking for it. Went shopping for dinner. Want to surprise him and apologize for fight. Bought fattening stuff he likes in case he wants to stay. Paid for it since I didn't actually ask if he wanted dinner. Didn't ask for money he owes me. Got back from store, Alex outside by his car, getting ready to leave. Seemed irritated. I mention dinner, hoping to entice him, but shut up when he says he's going home. Ate dinner alone. Opened wine I bought and drank the whole bottle myself. Cry.

### Sunday

Went shopping to cheer myself up. Saw great sweat-shirt but can't afford it due to going out and dinners and such. Bought shirt on sale for Alex. Matches his eyes. Hope he'll like it. Friend invited me to party at her place tonight. Said I could bring Alex but am scared to ask him and get turned down. Don't want to go alone because he gets jealous. Besides, he might want to get together to do something else. Mom called.

Cut her short because it was just when he's most apt to call me. Alex phoned an hour later; complained my line had been busy. I apologized; decided to keep line free in future in case he wants to reach me.

Those five diary entries put heft behind Gwen's decision to take back control of her life, but habits two years in the making rarely give up without a fight. She says that for her the solution was behavioral: "I had to start doing things that in the beginning bugged the hell out me, and just tolerate the flood of unpleasant feelings they generated. I started out with things I could do by rote, ones that didn't need much brains or heart." Reconnecting with her job was a top priority; unable to concentrate on her own demanding project, she asked junior staff members what they were working on and offered to help. Since the help they needed was straightforward, Gwen could focus long enough to provide it, thus propping up her diminished sense of self-worth. She cleared her desk of backlog, and her enthusiasm for her own project returned. Things were getting better.

Gwen took her health in hand. Although running her usual ten miles was out of the question, she forced herself to take a daily walk and fought off the desire to head home after five minutes to check her E-mail and phone messages. She still bought Cheetos and ice cream, but she added fruit to the mix. She couldn't go to a party, but she could invite her brother for dinner and be home, but not alone, should Alex drop by. She was still irritable on the phone with her mom, but she stopped apologizing to Alex for tying up the line. Soon Gwen could pick a film she wanted to see, invite Alex to join her, and if he didn't answer by the appointed time, make plans to go by herself or with a friend. When he sulked and complained that he had wanted to go, she told him he would have liked the film and that she had missed his company, leaving no room for another pointless argument that she would lose.

Gwen's small victories pumped up her self-esteem. They also had important implications for her immune system and, by extrapolation, for her physical and mental health. Should you think the leap from scenes avoided to the body's mechanism for fighting disease sounds far-fetched, cutting-edge research says otherwise. Readers up to curling their minds around a topic other than their immediate problems will find the research conclusions that follow rewarding; those whose brains are on overload may choose to fast-forward a couple of pages.

## HOW SCIENCE LEGITIMIZED
## THE MIND-BODY CONNECTION

As the early Greeks suspected, there is no separation between the mind and the body. Following in their footsteps several millennia later, Adelaide, engaged for fourteen years without a wedding ring in sight, stood on a Broadway stage in *Guys and Dolls* and belted out this home truth between sneezes and snuffles. The stress of unfulfilled expectations, resulting in a still-unadorned ring finger, had taken its toll: Adelaide had developed a persistent cold that refused to give way to the usual remedies of a spray or a shot. If you have ever blushed at a faux pas or a compliment, or endured a headache spiked by anger, or been plagued by worsening allergies in times of stress, the notion that emotions provoke bodily responses is hardly earth-shattering. Yet like a lot of home truths grounded in common experience, the mind-body connection languished in a New Age limbo for almost fifty years, thanks to science's insistence on hard research rather than anecdotal evidence.

Since then, a slew of technological advances and the interweaving of multiple medical disciplines—including endocrinology, biology, neurology, psychiatry, and immunology—have led to startling insights into the mind-body connection. When strung together, these disciplines spell psychoneuroimmunology, a new area of science that is already working its way from academia into the public sphere. Its jaw-breaking moniker expresses the interactive domains of psycho- (the mind and emotions), neuro- (the brain and central nervous system), and immunology (the body's cellular defenses against abnormal internal cells and external invaders such as bacteria or viruses). With its dawning, today's ubiquitous insistence on stress as the demon of contemporary life takes on a new meaning, not only for those who suffer from a wide range of physical illnesses far more serious than the common cold, but also for everyone deep in the stressful territory of depression fallout.

Dr. Esther Sternberg travels under the weighty twin titles of director of the Molecular, Cellular, and Behavioral Integrative Neuroscience Program and chief of the Section on Neuroendocrine Immunology and Behavior at the National Institute of Mental Health and the National Institutes of

Health, respectively. While she may look like a soccer mom, Dr. Sternberg presumably has little time for standing about on the sidelines. In *The Balance Within: The Science Connecting Health and Emotions,* she casts the immune system as the playing field on which our emotions and our body slug it out. Not long ago scientists thought that the immune response—a Star Wars attack on foreign invaders by the immune system's white cells—was self-regulating and could turn itself on and off autonomously without involving the brain. They based their assumption on the fact that the immune cells divided, multiplied, mobilized, and otherwise did their thing in laboratory petri dishes and test tubes with nary a brain in sight.

Detective work by Sternberg and others has established a dizzyingly complex communication system between the brain and the immune system that starts in the part of the brain called the hypothalamus, moves on to the pituitary gland, and then jumps all the way to the adrenals, two little glands perched on top of the kidneys, before rocketing back to the hypothalamus. In this cascading process, implanted in us eons ago as the lifesaving "fight or flight" response to danger and often termed the "stress response," adrenaline and cortisol course through the body, heightening our psychological and sensory awareness and speeding up our reactions. When the stressful experience is transitory, as in giving a speech, taking an exam, or narrowly being run over by a bus, our hormone-driven reaction to it serves us well; responses sharpened, we manage to deliver the speech, pass the exam, and leap out of the way of the bus. Once the fight-

or-flight hormones are no longer needed, the "on" button automatically switches off. If, however, the stressor is prolonged—as in a serious illness; fighting a war; prolonged sleep deprivation; starvation; or being trapped in a conflicted, frustrating, and unrewarding relationship—the on button jams; this allows cortisol, the most potent of the stress hormones, to flood and ultimately damage the heart and kidneys, among other organs.

If that were the sum total of the stress response, fallout sufferers could pat themselves on the back for being smart enough to grasp its rudiments, but there is more information to absorb. In addition to the hypothalamus-pituitary-adrenal axis described above, the ripple effect of stress also utilizes the central nervous system as a communications pathway between the immune system and the brain. When that crucial discovery was made some sixteen years ago, the door to a scientific basis for the mind-body connection opened wide, and psychoneuroimmunology (PNI to the cognoscenti) came into its own. Further research since then has established that the brain sends signals of stress to the immune system by involving the neurotransmitters—chemical messengers such as serotonin that are closely linked to human emotions—and that chemicals released by the immune system cells have an effect on the brain.

## SLIPPING FROM DEPRESSION FALLOUT INTO DEPRESSION

If Adelaide were singing her song today, she might be complaining of more than a cold, given the evidence hinting strongly at a close connection between a hyperactive immune system and depressive disorders. Researchers have uncovered an array of immunological changes associated with depression, among them a reduction in natural killer-cell activity, aka the white blood cells that mobilize to fight disease. They have also noted that depression is associated with changes in hormone levels akin to those found when the body is stressed, in particular, higher levels of the stress hormones cortisol, adrenaline, and noradrenaline. These interactions are so complex that careful scientists are unwilling to say whether depression or stress comes first, but the link between them clearly exists.

This link may explain why a significant number of Message Board veterans have slipped into a depression of their own. There are five possible explanations for this. The first is that those who have toppled over the edge into depression were born with a genetic vulnerability to the illness, passed along by a parent or grandparent, and that the chronic psychological stress under which they are laboring has triggered it. The second is that they may have been through a bout or two of mild depression in the past without attributing their lethargy, irritability, and changed sleeping and eating patterns to its proper cause, and that the current episode is just one in a series, exacerbated perhaps by circumstances.

The third possibility is that these fallouts have self-diagnosed their profound demoralization as depression, and that a well-meaning but inexpert general practitioner has mistakenly confirmed it. The fourth is that some Board visitors may have indulged in what academics call "assortative mating," a like-seeks-like theory suggesting that people inclined toward depression unconsciously seek one another out. Although this sounds bizarre, the phenomenon is sufficiently documented to deserve a modest place in the depression research literature. The fifth is that the brain, the central nervous system, and the immune system have reacted in concert to the emotional turmoil surrounding many fallout sufferers to induce an episode of depression.

Whichever explanation is correct, it is highly likely that stress played a leading role. Stress tolerance is personalized and probably genetically installed at birth; what overwhelms one person may leave another only temporarily shaken. What is sure is that loving someone with this illness is highly stressful and induces anxiety and demoralization, which in turn can sometimes for whatever reason(s) develop into the real thing. If you harbor any suspicion that you may have moved beyond depression fallout to depression, this is a prime opportunity to begin practicing the virtue of selfishness by putting your own problem above your partner's and checking it out with a skilled psychiatrist. Whether or not you are handed an antidepressant prescription, keep your focus firmly fixed on what you want and need. Sticking to that dictum is the surest way to reduce the psychological stress surrounding you to a manageable level.

## DEFINING AND SELF-DIAGNOSING PSYCHOLOGICAL STRESS

Depression fallout is rife with psychological stress, a working definition of which is cited by British behavioral biologist Paul Martin in *The Healing Mind: The Vital Links*

*Between Brain and Behavior, Immunity and Disease.* It is, Martin writes, "the state arising when the individual perceives that the demands placed on [him or her] exceed (or threaten to exceed) their capacity to cope, and therefore threaten their well being." Tucked inside that definition, warns Martin, is a crucial concept: Stress is as much a function of how we see the world as how the world really is, so taming it depends on how we appraise both the demands and our capacity to deal with them. In other words, stress, like beauty, is partly in the mind of the beholder. Pessimists fare badly. "Those of us whose world view is essentially pessimistic," he adds, "regarding our problems as pervasive, long lasting, insoluble and our fault, suffer worse damage from stress than those irritating optimists who always look on the bright side of life."

Even just-married couples undergo measurable stress when they talk about their relationship. One pair of PNI researchers at Ohio State University, having already established that women in poor-quality marriages tended to be in a worse state, both mentally and physically, than women whose marriages were thriving, assembled ninety newlywed couples, all of them healthy and happy. While each couple discussed the state of their brand-new union for half an hour, the researchers assessed their hormone levels, cardiovascular responses, and immune function using unobtrusive measuring techniques. Those couples that displayed the greatest hostility toward each other, even though it was only mild, had significantly lower scores on several measures of immune function. In addition, they experienced a temporary buildup of the stress hormones and an increase in blood pressure.

Given that even a brief post-honeymoon chat can generate stress, it's alarming to think how much bodily havoc goes on when one member of the relationship is depressed. Back in the mid-1980s, when nobody thought to scientifically measure stress levels, psychologist James C. Coyne assembled twenty-eight couples, seven with a depressed husband, seven with a depressed wife, and fourteen in which neither spouse was depressed. Each couple was invited to talk about a topic they considered a relevant relationship issue. When the allotted fifteen minutes had passed, the husband and wife were asked to rate their own and the other's coping strategies as either constructive (listening attentively), aggressive (name-calling and insulting one's partner), or withdrawal (sulking or pouting).

In Coyne's write-up of the experiment, aptly titled "Depression and Marital Disagreement: The Social Construction of Despair," he based his conclusions on the participants' reactions to and perceptions of each other rather than charting their biochemical reactions. The results showed that the partners of depressed spouses were just as upset in every way as their depressed husbands or wives; both were far more so than the depression-free couples. The depression-ridden couples were dissatisfied with their marriages and with their spouses' behavior in a conflict, though each judged his or her own behavior as blameless. At the end of their brief discussion, both partners were sad and angry; both experienced each other as hostile, competitive, mistrusting, and detached, as well as less agreeable, less supportive and encouraging, and less interested in becoming and feeling close.

If that list of adjectives sums up the state of your own and your partner's views of each other, you can safely count yourself among the severely stressed. Should you need further proof, turn on your computer, go to www.mayohealth.org, and take the Mayo Clinic's Stress Quiz, composed of ten questions ranging from "How often have you felt that you were unable to control the important things in your life?" to "How often have you felt that things were going your way?" After checking one of the suggested answers to each question—Never, Almost never, Sometimes, Fairly often, Very often—click the "Submit" button to receive your stress rating. That should persuade you that it's time to pay attention to yourself.

## TAMING YOUR STRESS RESPONSE

Getting a grip on stress requires more equipment than a pair of rose-colored glasses. This is because stress alters our perceptions, affecting not just our senses, but also memory, judgment, and behavior. Instead of trying to keep a stiff upper lip, try to recast the stress so that it is less threatening. Feeling that you have lost control over your life is tantamount to actually losing it. The Message Board teems with posts expressing the helplessness that overwhelms depression fallout sufferers. "I'm at a loss as far as my depressed husband is concerned," writes one. "I don't know how to handle him. I don't know how to cope except to be indifferent and ignore him. And to loathe him." More seasoned fallout sufferers know that it is impossible to ignore or be indifferent to a depressed person, even with the aid of blinders, earplugs, and a muzzle. And although sporadic fits of loathing can be temporarily invigorating, there are better ways to cope.

Lots of antistress remedies, from keeping a journal to thinking positive to relaxing in a lavender-scented bath with a novel, seem pitifully trivial compared to the magnitude of the problem. Who has time to take a brisk walk, tackle an overdue report in the office, or watch a funny movie when the major issues of life, such as love, commitment, and sharing the future with a spouse or lover, are in shambles? In fact, these seemingly mundane coping strategies (minus the bath and novel) turn up in the PNI research literature, couched more elegantly and grouped under headings like "behavioral interventions" or "mind-body technologies." Their purpose is to help you alter your perception of the problem so that it conforms to your coping abilities.

At first glance, the entries in Gwen's journal read more like a depression fallout anthem than an exercise in stress control. But spelling out the trivia of each day forced her to recognize that all her attempts to work, get organized, exercise, sleep more, and eat well kept giving way to a 24/7 preoccupation with her depressed boyfriend's moods and behavior. Instead of blaming herself for being unable to make everything right, she used the deceptively simple tactic of noting every action that compromised her own needs and countering it with positive behavior. This put her rather than the problem in charge. While it is unlikely that successful corporate managers keep a diary resembling Gwen's, they do practice a similar technique to escape from stress overload: Assess the problem, break it down to its most manageable parts, prioritize each component, and deal with them in order of urgency. All compulsive list makers know the satisfaction of crossing out even minor items accomplished; feeling in control is a potent antianxiety agent.

So is exercise. Health gurus have been touting its benefits for so long that it's easy to tune out their message and head for the couch. When that same message turns up in a tome devoted to PNI research, it's time to pay attention, especially when the author endearingly describes himself as a trifle pudgy and indolent. "I admit I would prefer not to dwell on this," writes Paul Martin, "but the truth must out." The truth is that in addition to its long-proven benefits in cardiovascular disease and the data linking it with improved health and longevity, even moderate exercise can elicit temporary increases in several key measures of immune function, including the number and activity of natural killer cells. But even if exercise brought no physical rewards whatsoever, the psychological benefits alone would make it worthwhile. Not only can it markedly improve mood; it can alleviate mild depression. People who exercise regularly and maintain a high level of physical fitness tend to experience less anxiety and depression; they sleep better, enjoy greater self-esteem, and feel more positive and in control.

## Gaining Control Through Relaxation

If the mere thought of an aerobics class induces indolence, consider relaxation instead. More than thirty years ago,

Dr. Herbert Benson trained some laboratory monkeys to lower their blood pressure by teaching them a few simple biofeedback principles. His students at Harvard Medical School urged their professor to investigate whether humans were as smart as laboratory primates. Using a group of experienced meditators as his first research subjects, Benson detected striking physiological changes as they shifted from everyday thinking into meditation and back again, among them a precipitous drop in the amount of a chemical called lactate in their bloodstream. High levels of lactate are associated with anxiety and panic attacks; low levels with a tranquil state of mind. Out of these findings grew Dr. Benson's "relaxation response," practiced by many cardiac-risk patients and, judging from the popularity of his many books about it, by numerous stressed-out devotees all over the world.

My guess is that Benson chose the term "relaxation response" over "meditation response" because the latter sounds like something only a Zen Buddhist can do. After three years of unsuccessfully trying to meditate at the end of my yoga class, I finally adopted a simple Benson-inspired routine that has saved my sanity in times of stress. This consists of lying down on my back, eyes closed, muscles relaxed (one by one if necessary), breathing slowly and deeply in and out six or eight times, and letting my mind float. If your mind is like mine, it will insist on gnawing at your problems, so keep it otherwise occupied by repeating a word or phrase ("freedom" works for me), concentrating on the flow of your breath, or conjuring up the image of a place you love. At first you'll be tempted to check your watch constantly, but within a couple of days your internal clock will set the alarm for twenty minutes. When you open your eyes, the world will look like a kinder, gentler place. Even more important, you will feel refreshed and full of energy and purpose.

## PUMPING UP YOUR SELF-ESTEEM

Loss of self-esteem is a prevailing problem for every traveler along the depression fallout continuum. Fallout sufferers are subjected to a steady stream of criticism and belittlement that efficiently clouds their view of themselves as admirable and viable human beings. Interactions with a depressed mate range from touchy to unbearable. When you offer love and affection, they are not returned. When you offer sympathy, you are told you don't understand what is wrong. When you offer support, you receive complaints that it is not enough, or not the right kind. Eventually, your internal mirror reflects your partner's distorted image of you. Blaming this on their depression is an objective and rational response, but objectivity and rationality are elusive commodities in such a situation. Instead of hoping they will fly in the window, look to your social support system for help.

Friends are the first line of defense for a battered ego, especially when they share your problem. As every user of the Message Board has discovered, empathetic support and understanding make intimates of disembodied posters who live half a world away. "What a sad commentary on my life," wrote one poster the day her bipolar husband took off after eating the breakfast she had cooked for him, "that I have to resort to posting my emotions on an Internet site for hundreds of strangers to read." "But you aren't talking to strangers," Guy replied. "You're talking to a lot of people in exactly the same situation who are your friends and care about you." This is why so many anguished visitors return over and over again to the Board.

The presence versus absence of social support has been thoroughly investigated by researchers; loneliness and isolation, they conclude, are unhealthy for mind and body. When you are under stress and down on yourself, you need friends, cyber or otherwise, to cheer you on, but the best ones to turn to are those who understand from their own experience what you are going through. A long outpouring by Board newcomer Confusedandscared hammers that truth home. Sandwiched between details of the couple's history—a husband of seven years who cycles in and out of depression yet refuses to seek treatment, threats of divorce because she's "so hard to get along with," vacations characterized by distance and unfriendliness—were reiterated self-accusations of weakness and selfishness. The Board immediately swung into action and responses flooded in from around the world, the first of them from Smiley: "Please hang in there!" she exhorted. "Everyone here will support you through this. I know how you feel—shaking, crying, can't eat, feeling so lost and alone. We all do. And we've been through the same desperateness you're feeling right now. It comes from seeing ourselves as helpless. I know it seems impossible, but try to step back and refocus on what you have control over."

"Focus on *you* right now," echoed Mike. "I think you're incredibly strong to have endured so much for so long without losing it completely and you should be really proud of that." "Take care of *yourself*," another ordered, and from Tia came instructions not to try to get through this alone: "Be good to yourself. Do things that you enjoy. See a therapist and come here often. We are here for you."

Widening your support system to include a psychotherapist is sound advice. Most fallout victims spend so much time and energy trying to get their depressed partners to seek therapy that they overlook their own need for it. Far from being self-indulgent, a weekly visit to an expert in short-term therapy will help you to order your priorities and to tackle those over which you have some control. A further advantage is that since you are paying for expert advice, you are more likely to listen and put it into practice; and because you are there for the express purpose of talking about yourself, there is no guilt attached to complaining about your depressed mate and outing your own virtues.

## ALTERNATIVES TO VENTING

"Just venting" is the heading used on the Message Board to introduce a detailed description of a depressed mate's latest iniquities. There is much to be said in favor of venting and the comforting me-too replies it provokes, but repeating the obvious leaves fallout victims languishing. The solution to moving past "Go" is to spend less time rehashing the latest scene and anticipating the next one, and more on anything and everything that gives you pleasure, whether it be sybaritic or intellectual. Tailor the following suggestions to your interests and keep reminding yourself that you feel as you do because of your partner's depression, not because you are at fault or lacking in some way.

Whatever you do well, do often. If you have any special talent in the arts, in sports, or in dealing with people, indulge it. Take a class in drawing, judo, or tap dancing; join an amateur singing or theatrical group; be a volunteer at a homeless shelter or the local hospital; teach an older friend how to use a computer. Listen to music, not as background noise but for the sheer joy of it; sign up for some lectures at a museum or community college; trace your genealogy, start a book club, experiment with baking, play poker with the guys and baseball with your kids. Buy some expensive soap and spend twice as long in the shower or bath; eat ice cream for breakfast; plant tulips in the yard. Get up and watch the sunrise. Your goal is to engage in pleasurable activities totally unrelated to your depressed person.

Stick to mastering skills that are within your reach. Do not attempt to learn Japanese or take up bungee jumping if you have no aptitude for languages and are scared of heights. Instead of a promise to run five miles a day, leave the car at home, walk to the office, and do errands on foot. Clean out the garage instead of painting the house. Decide to lose five pounds, not twenty, and to cut down a little on drinking and smoking rather than pledging to give them up. Read a good novel and put the book on quantum physics aside for the time being.

Do whatever reminds you that you are a good, intelligent, generous, responsible, and lovable person despite all evidence to the contrary offered by your partner. Spend time with people who like you as you are. To whatever extent possible, put some psychological and physical distance between you and your sad mate. If an hour of window shopping or coffee with a friend is all you have time for, grab the opportunity, but resist the temptation to make your problem the sum total of your conversation. Even the best of friends turn off after a while, especially if all they can do to help is to listen; nobody enjoys listening to a broken record and sooner or later their eyes will begin to glaze over. See friends instead as a window into a larger world, one not dominated by someone else's depression.

Make your own schedule instead of allowing your depressed partner to set it for you. That includes not sitting around waiting for a phone call that doesn't come. If your spouse or lover decides at the eleventh hour to stay home instead of going to the party, that does not mean you have to stay home, too. Warn anyone who extends an invitation to you as a couple that your partner may have to leave on a business trip, is subject to migraines, shows signs of developing the flu, or has a standing commitment for that evening, and go alone if necessary. Even though you think you may not feel like it, escaping the tension, even temporarily, will clear your mind and lighten your mood.

Apply yourself to your professional life, and take pride in accomplishments that lie outside the fixed parameters of your personal problems. A fair number of depressed people are workaholics, perhaps because working spares them the constant reminder that the rest of their life is in such disarray. In your case as well, work can have a beneficial effect. Instead of shutting down the computer at five o'clock sharp, stay later than usual in the office, even if only to shoot the breeze with your coworkers, or fabricate an excuse that justifies bringing home a bulging briefcase. It doesn't matter if there's not much in it of pressing import; polishing off a few overdue tasks will make you feel more organized and centered, and provides an alternative to unrewarding conversational efforts.

## Laughing Out Loud

Neither last nor least, indulge your sense of humor. Laughter is serious business for depression fallout sufferers, at the far end of the spectrum from the gut-churning anxiety and frozen-faced solemnity of stress. When I first began to monitor the Message Board, I noticed that responses to posts about the lighter side of life sometimes opened with LOL! and wondered what it meant; turns out it stands for laugh out loud. The welcome relief of even a small giggle is tangible; if you cannot find it within the situation, look elsewhere. Reading anything by Steve Martin or Woody Allen will cause an involuntary belly laugh. Watching the hapless Basil screw up in *Fawlty Towers,* the zany antics of the Monty Python gang, or the daily doings of Jerry Seinfeld and his loony friends will do the same for even the gloomiest fallout victims.

Daniel Goleman, writing in *Emotional Intelligence,*

reports on one of many experiments investigating the psychological benefits of a good laugh in solving problems that demand a creative solution. People who had just watched a video of television bloopers, the experiment showed, were better at solving a puzzle long used by psychologists to test creative thinking. In it people are given a candle, matches, and a box of tacks and asked to attach the candle to a corkboard wall so it will burn without dripping wax on the floor. Most people, says Goleman, fall into "functional fixedness," thinking about using the objects in only conventional ways. But those who had just watched the funny film were more likely to see an alternative use for the box holding the tacks, and so came up with the creative solution: tack the box to the wall and use it as a candleholder. Paul Martin recounts another video-watching experiment that demonstrates the biological advantages of humor. The blood hormone levels of participants were measured before and after being shown an amusing film; their post-video cortisol and adrenaline levels were significantly lower.

Now that you are in top mental and physical form, you are ready to face depression fallout's most serious problem: Where did your partner's love for you go, and what are you to do about it?

# 7

# I Love You,
# I Love You Not

Depression's cruelest trick is eroding love until even its memories fade and, like faces in old photographs, no longer seem familiar. That the illness can stifle the libido is accepted, but that it can also erase years of emotional intimacy surpasses understanding and is rejected by both partners. Each in his or her own way grapples with disbelief, allowing it to wedge its way between them. As their respective positions harden, so do their hearts. "I am trying to understand how, in just three months, I went from being my wife's 'only true love, forever,' to being responsible for all her misery," wrote one poster. "My husband took just a week to do the same," another replied.

Matters of the heart are conspicuously absent from research on depression and from the memoirs written by its sufferers. The best source of enlightenment is psychologists and therapists who are privy to the thoughts and feelings of depression and fallout sufferers alike, and an added assist comes from some famously melancholic poets, many of whom ended life by their own hand; the insights of both are offered in this chapter. If the suggested coping strategies are to succeed, fallout partners must bow to the incompatibility of depression and love. When the former enters, the latter is upstaged. Unless you take directorial control of the script, it will wind its way to an unhappy ending.

## QUESTIONS IN NEED OF ANSWERS

Depressed partners seem perplexed by love. Unable to assess its status, they flip back and forth from yes to no. Some stop on the negative and assert firmly that they are no longer attracted to their mate and take no pleasure in being with him or her, or that the relationship has simply run out of steam. Some go a step further, claiming that the cause of their depression is the strain of maintaining the facade of loving spouse, and that their mate's defensive, quarrelsome attitude makes it impossible to work things out. Others mutter vaguely of just not wanting to be married anymore, or, most puzzling of all, that they simply have no idea whether or not they are still in a state called love. Whatever their current assessment, it is likely to shift back and forth regardless of what has transpired in the interim, leaving fallout partners in constant fear that this day they will be told they are no longer loved.

The Message Board is incontrovertible proof of a lover's insatiable need to monitor, understand, and justify the state of the relationship. Newcomers' posts often start like posthumous love letters to a departed mate, reiterating the qualities that first bound them together. Believe me, they plead, my wife (or husband) is normally loving and affectionate, thoughtful and communicative, understanding and support-ive. After mourning the disappearance of these virtues, they pose a slew of questions arising from their mates' enigmatic utterances and behavior: What does she mean by saying that I deserve someone better? How can he claim to have no feel-ings for me anymore? How can she possibly view me as unsupportive and critical and defensive when I keep telling her how much I love her? How long can I go without any signs of affection and love from him? All these questions generate carbon-copy replies that commiserate but offer no solutions.

Veteran fallouts sound braver than newcomers, but their internal seismographs, too, tremble at the mysterious com-ings and goings of their partners' love. Commitment to the relationship leaves all of them feeling rejected and betrayed; surely, they think, depression alone cannot be the explana-tion. In search of I-love-you-too responses or confirmation of a beloved's alienation, they sift tirelessly through the rubble for other causes; finding none, they fall back on speculation. Sometimes their hypotheses, which range from gross selfish-ness to infidelity, are correct; depression can lead to both. But these are only clues to the prevailing cause. Accepting this requires a leap of faith and recourse to the few experts who have investigated why love and depression are such uneasy partners.

## ANHEDONIA: THE THEFT OF PLEASURE

Anhedonia is shorthand for "a marked loss of interest or pleasure in ordinary activities previously enjoyed" (often

with the addendum, "including sex"), an essential symptom in the diagnosis of depression. Ice cream and caviar
become as appealing as sawdust; the sensuousness of
spring in all its budding glory doesn't tweak a response;
neither Miles Davis nor Mozart can perk up anhedonic
ears. Everything previously counted on to pleasurably stir
memories and spark anticipatory gusto fails to work its
usual magic. Nonprofessionals assume this is part and par-
cel of the social withdrawal and lassitude that mark this
illness. Depression sufferers often attribute it to boredom
and being in a rut. Inertia of the senses leaves a vacuum
that cries out to be filled; breaking the confining mold of
routine with novelty and experimentation, sloughing off
the old and embracing something new and different are
classic come-hithers to the dissatisfied.

Psychiatrist Peter Kramer says he could fill his entire
practice with cases of falling out of love, so common is this
complaint, and starts looking for evidence of depression
when he hears it. His view is that such cases are prime
examples of anhedonia, a biological relative, or even an
equivalent of depression. In his book about divorce,
*Should You Leave?* Kramer sketches a first visit scenario
starring a patient who has come for confirmation that the
marriage is over, and who insists that the spouse once
cherished, although for reasons now forgotten, stirs not a
glimmer of love. Kramer recognizes this perspective as the
product of an altered mood, but to the patient it is utterly
convincing: The love is truly dead and gone.

The patient rejects the proffered opinion that anhedonia is the cause, insisting that depression has absolutely

nothing to do with the situation because he (or she) *does* look forward to activities and *does* takes pleasure in them. He enjoys hanging out with old friends, for example, and is certainly capable of passion since he has fallen in love with a fascinating new woman. But Kramer knocks down these arguments. His patient doesn't find real pleasure when he drinks and gambles with buddies, only compulsive stimulation that offers momentary escape from pain and emptiness. "And what are we to make of your readiness to withdraw from contact with your children, whom you say you adore?" he asks. The truth is that "You can no longer feel pleasure in any sphere. When you report that you enjoy yourself in this or that context, it is because you no longer remember what pleasure is."

Dr. Kramer is entirely unsympathetic to his patient's current passion for the unencumbered someone, whom he characterizes as liking action, complications, intrigue, and legally attached spouses. "When you say that you need her [or him] to arouse you, you're saying that your hedonic capacity is turned way down low so that it takes enormous stimulation to move you at all." Once his patient's family turmoil is resolved by separation or divorce and he is on his own, warns Kramer, the romance will not last a month.

Even if this warning were pasted on the bathroom mirrors of all depressed mates who have "fallen out of love," and even if Dr. Kramer's consulting room were big enough to accommodate them, many subsequent visits, combined with antidepressant medication, would be necessary to shake their anhedonic view of the relationship. The stubbornness the depressed display in defending their perspective is a further testament to depression's guile. When they agree to see a doctor or therapist it is not because they think they are wrong but to give the appearance of being reasonable. Not all psychiatrists and psychotherapists are as enlightened and persistent as Dr. Kramer, who hates the insidiousness of mood disorder as a cancer surgeon hates the insidiousness of cigarettes.

Some therapists bolster the patient's belief that the underlying issue is indeed an unhappy relationship, and that depression is its product, not its cause. An example of this showed up on an Internet Web site that invites questions about mental health, including relationships, answered by a nameless entity called Psych Online. Under the heading "Wife says she doesn't love me," the writer asks what he can do to help his wife get better (she is already on antidepressant medication), and says he will wait until that goal is accomplished before addressing her I-no-longer-love-you declaration. Psych Online is "curious" about the man's conviction that waiting is the right decision because, he says, marital problems may indeed be causing her disaffection. "Perhaps you need to listen more fully and more deeply to her and assume nothing except that she means what she says and has good reasons for saying it." A similar psychotherapeutic approach may explain an E-mail received from a Message Board visitor. Opening with a synopsis of her lover's history of depression, for which he had recently been visiting a therapist, the writer explains that on Sunday her lover told her he couldn't imagine life without her and looked forward to their marriage. On Tuesday, following an appointment with the therapist, he announced that he had said this only out of guilt. As already noted, the depressed present their perspective with conviction, and even therapists can be conned into accepting it.

## CREATIVE GENIUS ON THE COUCH

Many creative geniuses have been subject to severe depressive illness and have articulated their loveless pain for all the world to hear. In Kay Redfield Jamison's study of the link between depressive illness and the artistic temperament, *Touched with Fire,* the diaries, correspondence, and works of the poets and other artists she quotes read like transcriptions of a therapy session taped for public consumption. Scattered throughout are admissions of depression's dual assault upon pleasure and moral judgment.

William James (all but one of whose four siblings inherited their father's depression) evinces what Peter Kramer would know to be anhedonia: "Unsuspectedly from the bottom of every fountain of pleasure . . . something bitter rises up: a touch of nausea, a falling dead of the delights, a whiff of melancholy, things that sound a knell, for fugitive as they may be, they bring a feeling of coming from a deeper region and often have an appalling convincingness." Samuel Johnson refers to his melancholy as "that depression of mind which enchains the faculties without destroying them, and leaves reason the knowledge of right without the power of pursuing it." Robert Lowell equates his black moods with a withering of the senses, and says of one collection of poems that "[m]ost of the best poems [in it], the most personal, are gathered crumbs from the lost cake. I had better moods, but the book is lemony, sourced, and dry, the drought I had touched with my own hands." What rings throughout these quotes is the authors' impotent frustration; they know that something is grievously wrong, but are powerless to redress it.

Lord Byron, whose history of marriage and illicit affairs paralleled his gyrations between mania and despair, counted himself among "an order of mortals on the earth, who do become old in their youth . . . [and] die of withered, or of broken hearts." The poet once wrote to a friend that he was "indeed very wretched . . . all places are alike, I cannot live under my present feelings, I have lost my appetite, my rest, & can neither read write or act in comfort." Jamison likens the poet's famously mercurial temperament—described by Byron as "a war, a chaos of the mind"—to a field of tectonic plates clashing and grating against one another and notes that for virtually all his life, Bryon engaged in "a consuming civil war within his own mind, which, then convulsing outward, at times was waged as anything but civil war on the people and world around him."

Even the Jekyll-Hyde phenomenon, characterized by Dr. Jamison as the gap that frequently exists between public appearance and private despair, shows up in her study. The Austrian composer Hugo Wolf seems almost to have been addressing an audience of fallout partners when he wrote, "I appear at times merry and in good heart, talk, too, before others quite reasonably, and it looks as if I felt, too, God knows how well within my skin; yet the soul maintains its deathly sleep and the heart bleeds from a thousand wounds." If he or she could find the words, your partner would tell you the same and echo "amen" to these eloquent expressions of anhedonia by some of the world's most gifted men and women.

Not long ago an unsung poet, who also suffers from depression, sent me an E-mail about losing her husband's love: "When he told me that he loved me I thought he must be lying because how could anyone love me. I hated myself with a passion and couldn't even look in the mirror anymore." She accepted his decision to move out, but has since gone on antidepressants; now "free from the 'demons' inside my head," she longs for his return. One hopes she has shared with him the following lines from her poem titled "At Last."

Too many years spent
in the shadow of life.
Too long endured the pain
of a heart bleeding with sadness.
Shallow breath,
no longer the feeling of
love, of life—
walking the path of death.
At last the spell is broken,
and with every new beam of light
the decision is made
to choose love,
to choose life once again.

## THE DEPRESSION SUFFERER'S DARKEST SECRET: "I DO NOT LIKE MYSELF"

Less eloquent sufferers forego phrases like "a falling dead of the delights" and state their plight bluntly, but the feelings expressed are the same. "I'm miserable, rotten, and lousy," writes one depressed wife on an Internet message board called Depression Forum. "I feel like I'm invisible in all aspects of my life, inadequate and unappreciated. My husband does nothing but criticize my every move, and I'm so tired of living with a man who obviously doesn't even like me. No one seems to have time for a pathetic person like me. I could disappear and nobody would notice." Her partner quite likely tells her that he loves her and makes all manner of accommodations to show his support and concern, may even be communicating his side of the story on the fallout Message Board. What is most notable about this post, however, is the lethal combination of self-denigration and self-pity it reveals.

The depressed think very poorly of themselves. The torrent of criticism directed at partners is the overflow from the reservoir of self-hatred in which their psyches soak. Feeling unworthy, stupid, inept, ugly, emotionally bereft, and unlovable, they are angry with themselves for being so lacking in every way, and they get angry with you, the person who knows them better than anyone, for not accepting what is obvious to them. This is not a secret the depressed choose to shout from the rooftops, but when they do, their partners have trouble accepting what they hear as the truth and dismiss it as a manipulative attempt to wring sympathy where none is deserved. As one frustrated poster put it, "This is such a 'me' illness. Everything is always about them, they're always in such pain, blah, blah, blah, they never think of the pain they're causing us." The observation is partially true; the depressed are at the center of their universe, but the centrist position they assume robs them of a hiding place from the judgments they make about themselves. When they tell you that you deserve someone better, it is the product of introspection.

That old homily, "You can't love others if you don't love yourself," is a fitting epitaph for the depression sufferer's intimate relationships. Elizabeth's lengthy tale of sorrow documents her marriage to a man she has known since junior high school. For eight years they had counted on spending their life together, but as the long awaited wedding day grew closer, her fiancé began to talk of "needing space," yet at the same time sent her flowers with notes of "love forever." They saw a couples therapist, who wisely diagnosed her fiancé's hesitation as probable depression, an illness that runs in his family; after several months of Prozac, they went to the altar a contented couple. Soon afterward, her husband stopped taking his medication and discontinued therapy on the grounds that love would solve any problems, but devotion failed. He emulated many other depressed spouses, returning home late and often drunk, refusing to eat dinner with his wife, and unwilling to make weekend plans; six months later Elizabeth moved back in with her parents. Her husband, Elizabeth reports, says that although he does love her, he cannot make her happy and wants her to move on, that he is truly sorry for this and that she deserves someone much better than he. Sometimes he hugs her and clings to her; sometimes he withdraws completely because, he explains, being with her reminds him of all the pain he is causing her.

Elizabeth's post drew many replies from others whose experiences duplicated hers in many respects and a chorus of entreaties to take care of herself, to put her needs first, to see a psychotherapist, and to recognize that she can do nothing to change her husband. So accustomed are frequent Board visitors to the loss of love that not one response commented on her husband's declarations of love and his claim that he was unworthy of her. Had they known the following story about Richard O'Connor and his wife Robin, they would have been more hopeful.

## A RELATIONSHIP BIG ENOUGH TO ENCOMPASS DEPRESSION

Richard O'Connor, introduced in Chapter 4 as the author of *Undoing Depression* and an admitted depression sufferer, has a successful marriage even though in many respects he bears a close resemblance to the depressed partners described on the Message Board. As a clinical social worker, Richard had seen many men and women whose lives were ruined by their depression and hoped that the book, addressed to fellow sufferers rather than to their mates, would help readers avoid a similar fate.

Even though Richard had experienced an episode of depression during college, and even though he was already taking medication to counteract insomnia when he began writing and added Prozac to bolster his energy, he told me that he hadn't thought of himself as depressed, just as a low-energy person who needed a boost. But writing about other people's depression forced the author for the first time to apply its diagnostic criteria to himself. He knew the value of good counseling; his mother committed suicide when Richard was only a teenager, and he had years of ongoing psychotherapy under his belt. During a weekly therapy session, Richard asked if the therapist thought it was possible that he, like his prospective readers, could perhaps have depression, to which the therapist replied, "Are you kidding, of course you do!"—another spectacular example of depression blindness.

That Richard's depression had not already undermined his marriage was due to the union's underlying strength. Both Richard and Robin grew up in troubled environments and sought the terra firma of a love they could always count on. When they got married they made a pact that their relationship would be a lifelong commitment, a promise that sustained them even as Richard played the depressed spouse role in all its destructive glory. "Depression has a lot to do with shame," he told me. "Inflicting that shame on someone else helps because it makes you feel powerful and in control. Anger makes you feel like you're the boss, at least in the short run, although in the long run it drives others away." Although functional during his office hours, Richard withdrew from his family when he came home. His way of handling his guilt was to do things "for" Robin and the kids, like building a sundeck they hadn't asked for, then feeling victimized out there in the heat. "I'd come back inside grouchy and have a couple of stiff drinks to make myself feel better. I ruined a lot of weekends that way," he said with a rueful smile.

Although medication has helped Richard, like all savvy depressives, he knows antidepressants can't do the job alone. He works to keep the marriage healthy by monitoring himself continually, "like an alcoholic in recovery. I need to be clear on what makes me feel good or bad." He is careful not to isolate himself, watches his alcoholic intake, and capitalizes on opportunities for having fun, as well as taking generic precautions such as exercising, eating right, and getting enough sleep. Richard knows that he fits his description of a depression sufferer as "withdrawn, shut off, and totally self-involved." The depressed, he explained, put up an impenetrable wall and feel both beyond help and undeserving of their partner's love. "When the partner asks, 'How do you feel, what are you thinking?' we haven't an answer, even for ourselves. No spouse can understand how much depression affects thinking; it's beyond them. When you're full of self-loathing and they're telling you how crazy they are about you, there's a huge disconnect."

Robin's contribution to their marital pact includes understanding, and sympathetically tolerating, the behavioral exigencies of her husband's depression. When questioned about how he thought Robin was able to go on loving him despite what she calls his "looks of condescension and disdain" and his hypercritical attitude, Richard seemed taken aback, and then replied that he thought it was because she has always believed in him, "in my basic desire to do the right thing." Perhaps, too, although Robin cannot fully comprehend what lies behind the wall, she knows a great deal about depression and has learned how to make room in their marriage for her husband's illness. She is, Richard says, good at coaxing him to "come out and play in a gentle way," and doesn't tease him about being grumpy. Instead, Robin creates opportunities for Richard to have fun with the family, but keeps arrangements flexible because she understands the demands of his changing moods.

Key to the couple's success is a system of signals devised to help Robin distinguish between Richard's differing needs. "Right now I just need you to listen to me" and "Right now I have a problem I need you to help me with" are, he explains, two entirely different appeals for help, and when Robin occasionally misreads them, it upsets him. Richard's advice to fallout spouses is to be attuned to the distinction, and to just listen without speaking when your partner feels like opening up. But you can't plan ahead for this, he warned; it has to happen at the moment your depressed partner wants to talk.

Asked how Robin dealt with his self-denigration, Richard said that she tells him not to be too hard on himself. And does that help? "Not at the time," he replied, "but it's the right thing to say. Just go on saying it even though it doesn't ring true to your depressed partner." Among his other tips for fallout spouses: Educate yourself about the illness so that you can disengage from it without disengaging from the person. Accept that you cannot change the way your depressed mate thinks and use boundaries to put a rein on hurtful behavior. Be polite, caring, and as affectionate as your partner will permit, and learn how to protect yourself when the going gets very tough.

## THE OTHER MAN OR WOMAN

At the heart of Richard O'Connor's advice is unquestioning support and unquestioning love, a difficult prescription to follow. This requires that you accept those occasional glimpses of the person with whom you fell in love as real and the stranger as a chimera. Faith is put to the test when an affair is suspected; in truth, many spouses and lovers suspected of straying are either sitting alone in their cars or trying to pretend they are having fun drinking with their office buddies. Those who do indeed track down an unencumbered person satisfy several needs, among them confirmation that someone out there deems them attractive and alluring. You cannot meet that need because of the perceived disconnect between your declared devotion and their unworthiness. Furthermore, the new person doesn't keep asking how they are feel, or get on their back about undone chores, or expect children to be helped with homework and cheered at soccer games, or complain about their drinking. And what better than novelty with a dash of intrigue to jump-start a flagging libido? An illicit lover may be more willing to accept sex without the emotional intimacy expected by a long-term partner, but even though the new relationship is less entangling and has no past to demand comparison, the passion is a distraction and will not last because it cannot withstand the anhedonia at its core.

The above are explanations, not excuses. Most depressed men and women ride out their illness without succumbing to temptation; infidelity, like physical violence directed at others, is within the depressive's control, but the temptation to thwart anhedonia is very strong. The standard excuse is that the affair doesn't mean anything because it has nothing to do with love. In the case of the depressed, this excuse is more closely linked to deadness of the heart than to waning of affection for the spouse. Some cheating partners have told their mates that the man or woman in question is a fellow sufferer of depression and "understands" them, suggesting there is a misery-loves-company factor in play.

The pain depressed partners cause is no less real for having sprung from angst, and partners can hardly be expected to endure it passively. Dodging direct confrontation, a number have composed letters to their cheating spouses and put them on the Board with an invitation to comment. The letter Christopher wrote to his depressed wife and shared with the Board was part excellent model, part example of what not to say. The opening paragraph exactly suited the couple's current situation: "Our marriage is broken. I honestly believe that it can be repaired if we're both willing to do the necessary hard work." One hopes, however, that he edited out, "I will understand if you find it easier to move on and try again with someone else, a decision I wouldn't be able to respect, but it would be completely understandable." Depressed partners need to know that they are cherished. Christopher's final paragraph, which opened with "I do not hate you for this," was intended to counter his wife's complaints that he was too understanding, too free of anger. But Christopher's letter is so anger-free that it might well give the impression that he was proposing a reconciliation out of good manners and a sense of responsibility.

When a fallout partner decides on written rather than verbal communication, it is wise to write three or four different versions, put them away for a week or so, and then pick the one that best reflects his or her true thoughts and feelings. Non-depressed mates who are seeing a therapist could ask the therapist for editing suggestions. The advantage is that the therapist knows your side of the story and how it is affecting your feelings and sense of self. In one such instance, a therapist blue-penciled out a dozen dangerous buzzwords such as *coward, ashamed,* and *appalled.* The resulting "cool" letter produced apologies and opened the way to a productive talk.

## DEPRESSION AND THE SEX DRIVE

The majority of depression sufferers have a diminished interest in sex, and most antidepressant medications cause sexual dysfunction in as many as 80 percent of users. Few people tell the truth about their sexual dysfunction, even in anonymous questionnaires, and doctors follow a "Don't ask, don't tell" policy, so it is not surprising that the depressed and their partners, too, shy away from frank discussion of this problem. Silence in the face of persistent disinterest in making love, or of failure to achieve erection or to reach orgasm, exacerbates the loss of intimacy. Brian, whose wife has withdrawn from him and refuses to talk about it, feels abandoned, "kind of on the outside looking in. I know a relationship isn't all about sex, but it certainly can be fun, and sexual identity is an important part of one's psyche."

The sexual double whammy has psychiatrists and pharmaceutical companies scratching their heads. At present, there are only three antidepressants, Wellbutrin, Effexor, and reversible MAOIs—called Manerix and Aurorix, but unavailable in the United States—that appear to permit most users to have enjoyable sex; Serzone and Remeron have been reported by some users as satisfactory in this respect. The worst offenders are those most frequently prescribed, including Prozac, Zoloft, and Paxil, but it is important to remember that everyone is different; a drug that adversely affects one person's libido may leave another's intact. There are counteractive measures, not all of them safe or reliable, such as foregoing antidepressants for twenty-four hours before having sex, called taking a "drug holiday," or switching to another drug. When invited to do so, knowledgeable physicians will discuss the options. These may include adding a second antidepressant or one of the reportedly helpful herbal extracts; Viagra helps many men and clinical trials with women are ongoing. Pretending that there is no sexual problem by keeping secrets from doctors and from partners is the worst possible approach.

A group of experts assembled by the National Depressive and Manic-Depressive Association offers non-depressed partners a fourfold solution. Maintain a physical connection in an unthreatening way by just cuddling and hugging—a tactic many Board fallouts have tried, only to be met with flinching, as though their touch were repellent. Be patient and let your mate know you'll be there when he or she feels ready. Share your feelings with him or her. This step is less difficult than it seems. The trick is to avoid saying anything that might sound to depressed ears like criticism; let your partner know that you're concerned about the changes in your shared sex life and that you miss physical closeness. This works best if you stick to "I" statements—"I miss your touch," "I feel rejected and unattractive when you don't want to have sex"—rather than casting the issue in terms of his or her attitude and performance. The fourth and final suggestion, by far the most problematic, is not to take it personally.

## "Don't Take It Personally"

Message Board posters do take personally the absence of affection and sexual interest; how could they not? One observed that just because you are being ground up in the cogs of a depression machine that barely knows you're there doesn't make it impersonal. "I'm not some generic 'loved one,' I'm me," he pointed out. "Okay, I accept that my depressed wife isn't maliciously focused on hurting me, but that perspective ignores the fact that I *am* being hurt." Another poster chimed in that she had asked her husband for something to go forward on, even a crumb. "He looked at me as though I were crazy and then said that nothing had changed, but *everything* has changed," she said.

Asking your depressed partner if he or she loves you requires a new dictionary of love. The odds of receiving a clear, affirmative response are slim; more likely, the reply will be couched in the idiom of the depressed. "I'm still here, aren't I?" means "If I didn't love you I would have left by now"; "I know, you keep telling me that" is the equivalent of "I told you I don't deserve you"; a muffled "Thanks" can be interpreted as "Hang in there, I need you."

To continue chiseling away at a cold exterior in the hope of extracting something more positive is a deathblow to self-esteem. Those who have attempted to initiate sex often meet with rejection, and as a result feel undesirable and ashamed. One wife described her self-esteem as "so low I felt like I was crawling on the ground under an ant" and wondered why she kept letting herself get hurt over and over again. Peter, recounting his attempts to just get close to his depressed wife and prove to her that everything was okay, said that her repeated rejection caused him to question not his manliness, but his worth as a supportive and loving spouse. Many are left feeling incomplete and as though their feelings were of no consequence to their partners.

There is no simple solution that will work for every fallout partner, but Gwen, in need of confirmation that her love is returned, has come up with one that is helpful to her. Instead of saying "I love you" and then waiting breathlessly, only to experience another whop of disappointment when the reply is, "Uh-huh," Gwen suggests you ask your partner cheerfully and matter-of-factly, "Do you love me?" If the answer is "I don't know," her recommended response is "Well, I hope you do. I would like that." If the depressed partner delivers what the Board calls the whole blah-blah-blah speech—"I don't know what I feel, I'm dead inside, I don't feel much of anything"— recognize that they are talking about themselves, not about you. When her boyfriend gives that speech, Gwen lets him wind down and then says, "I understand what you're saying and I know it's hard for you to try to answer me directly. But it would make me happy to know that you *think* you do love me, and I'm asking you to tell me now if that is true." Notice that this conversational strategy relies on lots of "I's" and sympathetic listening to cushion the request for a direct answer. It avoids giving the impression of intense emotional neediness on Gwen's part—which might be threatening to her mate—and requires only a statement of fact, not a heavy conversation. Fallouts who give this a try may get what they are looking for; even if it's not entirely satisfying, it is far more rewarding than just ignoring what's going on in the bedroom.

Men posting on the Board have been less forthcoming than women in airing their thoughts about a partner's diminished interest in making love, but a few who have opened up report being confused when she returns cuddles with cuddles and then turns away if they try to initiate sex. Women as a whole place as much importance in bed on affectionate displays as on good sex, so cuddling without trying to take it further is a good way for men to maintain emotional intimacy with their depressed wife or lover. When men are depressed, fallout mates should reassure their partner that while they enjoy having sex and share his frustration that it's not working easily right now, this does not mean that they think less of him because of it. In either case, don't avoid talking about the obvious; depressed mates need reassurance even though they often appear to reject it.

## A Word About Pornography and Substance Abuse

Fallout wives report acute distress over their partners' sudden interest in porn. Anita speaks for many of them in saying that her husband's preference for visiting Internet sex sites rather than initiating intimacy with her is crushing, and admits she would like to receive even a fraction of what "those computer babes" are getting. Yet in most instances, turning to porn addresses a need that has little to do with a partner and is a comparatively benign substitute for extramarital sex. Think of the depressed as frustrated drivers who repeatedly press the accelerator of a stalled car; they go on gunning the engine in hope of signs of life. Porn offers a way for the depressed to feel momentarily alive by pushing mental buttons that have little to do with real intimacy.

Though it is upsetting to come upon a hidden stash of *Playboy* magazines or to discover that the computer is bookmarked for quick access to Internet sex sites, fallout partners would do well to accept these as straightforward attempts to prod the libido. Instead of feeling demeaned and threatened, consider the distinct possibility that the porno photographs, X-rated videos, and sexual chat rooms are preludes to performing well in your bed. Indeed, one expert on sex and depression suggests to her patients that they invite their partners to watch those videos with them.

Alcohol is no help to sex, but it does temporarily turn down the level of depressive pain. Increased use of alcohol and drugs is not on the official symptoms list, but they often go hand in hand with depression. Most doctors allow moderate drinking for patients on antidepressants, although there are exceptions to this rule, notably when a partner is bipolar. The problem with drinking and drugging is that there is no end to the pain, and reaching escape in the form of near-oblivion becomes the preeminent goal. Fallout partners who have good reason to believe that drug taking and drinking are out of control can exert some influence by drawing a boundary, but like all substance abusers, the depressed substance abuser will overstep it. Asking him or her to moderate their drinking in your presence is a more practical solution than trying to ban it completely.

# 8

# Mending or Breaking
the Bond

The Message Board is an archive of hopes realized, abandoned, and in abeyance. Encouraged by the empathetic support it offers, posters have been able to express the tangle of thoughts and emotions that ultimately will lead to agonizing decisions: Can this bond be mended, or is it broken beyond repair? Is it selfish and unfair to abandon someone who suffers from this illness? Can mutual trust be rebuilt? Is love enough to warrant yet another try? What will this mean for the children? Answers fall into no easily discernible pattern, governed as they are by the many factors in play. The temperament of each partner, the relationship's past history, the severity of the illness, and immediate issues such as children, finances, and the emotional support available from family and friends all clamor for attention.

Every non-depressed partner facing the leave-or-stay dilemma must put each of these factors on the scales and tally the sum of their collective weight. Both Penny and

Sam came to the Board in its earliest days, but arrived at differing conclusions, hers to stay and his to leave. Both chose the right path; neither found it easily, but they are following their respective courses with confidence and the serenity that comes from honest self-examination. Both believe they have grown through their experience and now have a deeper understanding of themselves and of what is important to them. Their stories serve to illustrate that there is no generically "correct" decision or overriding moral construct to be followed in such situations, only individual truths arrived at through hard work and not a little pain.

The decision-making process is made all the more difficult by the clash of love and anger. Trying to make sense out of these conflicting emotions, all the while hoping beyond hope that the "real" partner will emerge triumphant and that love will prevail, sends resolve into a tailspin. Few fall-out partners freely embrace separation or divorce; circumstances beyond their control force an unwanted choice upon them. When a poster admitted that it would be easier to deal with her spouse's death than his depression and consequent rejection of her, a dozen replies urged her not to feel guilty for thinking that way. "Death isn't so personal as divorce," said one. "If my husband were to die, I wouldn't have the pain of thinking he didn't love me anymore. I wouldn't feel that I have failed as a wife and as a woman." Another spoke for many in expressing his anger at a mate who, ignoring his love and commitment to their marriage, has chosen to leave him for a man she has known only six months. "I am the scapegoat for my wife's inner turmoil and her refusal to face it honestly. Death is much kinder," he wrote, "it doesn't taunt or bully those who are left behind."

Dissolution of a marriage or a long-lasting relationship, always a painful process, is even more heartrending for fallout partners. Knowing that a treatable illness is the main obstacle to mending the bond makes coming to a firm decision very difficult, but there are signals that hint at the most likely outcome. Where to look for them and how to interpret their meaning is clarified by reviewing the stream of serial updates posted by Penny and by Sam over time: two stories similar in all but their ending.

## GOING . . . GOING . . . GONE?

The episode of depression that brought Penny to the Board was her husband's second; the first, which had occurred four years earlier, predated her knowledge of its cause and also the birth of a daughter. This time she had some inkling of the underlying cause when her husband once again announced that he didn't know if he wanted to be married, didn't know if he still loved her, and treated her accordingly. Penny's posts over a year track all five stages of depression fallout. Although her husband had agreed to see a marriage counselor with her, the sessions were a failure. Not only did Penny's husband deny depression and insist he had nothing more serious than a sleep disorder, he added that his self-esteem was healthy, that he was not the cause of his wife's unhappiness, and that he had no guilt at all. When the therapist suggested that perhaps he was pushing Penny away because he felt unworthy of a good relationship, he answered with a resounding negative. The suggestion that he see a therapist on his own met a similar fate. Tired, as Penny said, of the games, the lying, the whole ball of wax, she told him one June day that she was ready to file for divorce.

An added worry for Penny was the lesson their young daughter might draw from observing her mother's seeming tolerance of emotional abuse. Penny feared that in appearing to accept her husband's ugly behavior at home, she was conveying a dangerous message about marriage and love, and that the girl might grow up believing that it's normal to live with a man who not only lies but also continually hurts the woman he supposedly loves most in the world. "I wish I could go that extra mile, but I'm losing myself, and my daughter is suffering," wrote Penny after setting herself a deadline: one last weekend devoted to trying to penetrate her husband's defenses, during which she would make clear her willingness to stay if he were willing to get the help he needed to change. Facing up to the strength of his denial, on Monday she packed a month's supply of clothes and moved with her daughter to her parents' home seven hundred miles away.

The hoped-for changes came in fits and starts, and the thirty-day deadline was extended to two months. The first big crack in the wall came when her husband went to a psychiatrist for his "sleep disorder" and was prescribed an antidepressant—not, as it ultimately developed, the right one for him, but effective enough to give him a more flexible perspective on what divorce and the loss of his daughter meant to him. His promise to "work on their problem" was insufficient reason for her return; it was a promise she had heard many times before and only served to intensify her anger and resentment. Penny wanted harder evidence of good intentions, something more tangible than her husband's stated wish to remain a family and to try to allow her to get close to him. Although he continued to dodge responding to the "needs" list she had presented to him— sharing, friendship, trust, and love—his telephone calls became more frequent, and Penny began to see a man in pain and confusion, frightened by the dawning realization that the crunch had come.

By mid-August Penny reported to the Board that her husband now sounded deflated but rational, no longer "the monster I've been living with for so long." When he began seeing a therapist, Penny invited him to come for a weekend so that they could talk at length, and the visit was a success. He brought with him her list of needs and item by item told her specifically what he would do to meet them. And he told her that he loved her and begged for another chance to prove it. All three of them returned home together, and the real work of restoring their marriage began, a work still in progress but nearing completion now, two years after the dam broke.

Sam posted a warning about the state of his marriage under the heading "Going . . . going . . . ?" and then, three months later, announced its denouement with "Gone!" His explanatory post was brief, citing the toxicity of life at home and his current wish to crawl into a hole and pull it in after himself. He had hoped that by refusing to leave as asked, there would be time to talk things out, but when his wife advanced upon him with a potato peeler, shouting that he better leave before one of them got hurt, he packed up his life in boxes and fled to a rented two-room apartment. "I still love my wife with all my heart, but if she is unwilling to accept me and my love there isn't much else I can do right now except look out for myself," he wrote.

In time Sam found some blessings to count: He's no longer forever waiting for his wife to explode; the children, both in their teens, drop by most days after school to reassure him of their love; his father has been less judgmental than anticipated, has encouraged Sam to talk about his feelings, and has offered good advice and much support. "I guess," Sam wrote one day, "that I am halfway through the process so many of you describe: short-lived relief; incredible sadness, self-blame, and regret; denial of what has happened and sympathy for my wife; gut-wrenching loneliness; obsessive replaying of every argument and mistake; anger and, finally, peace. I feel such incredible sadness and emptiness. While I can think about this with some objectivity, the emotional part is just ripping me up. It's so hard to believe that someone who is supposed to love you can be so cruel, so cutting, and so blind to the truth."

Sam is once again seeing the psychotherapist who helped him through previous bad times, but "the emotional journey will be my own. It will be painful, but I will survive." He had been waiting, he says, for the magic-wand effect by which his wife would suddenly wake up free of depression and in love with him again. Now convinced that this will never happen, he has begun unpacking the boxes and starting to put his life back in order, at least that part of it which he can control. "I had thought of this apartment as a temporary refuge. It's not. . . . It's home now, and I will live here alone and get well."

## SIGNALS AND WHAT THEY PORTEND

In the months preceding their respective decisions, Sam and Penny were living under very similar circumstances. Their depressed partners, in denial about their illness and the havoc it was causing, were using them as targets for their own feelings of resentment, anger, and inadequacy; their horizons were limited, extending no further than the pain of the moment. If it were possible to calculate the dimensions of love, Sam's and Penny's would have the same width, breadth, and depth; neither lacked purpose, and both had children to factor into the equation. The desire to preserve their marriages was equally strong. The reasons why one survived and one ended may lie in the timing and intensity of the illness from which their partners suffered. Perhaps if Sam's wife had in the past gone through an overt episode of depression that jeopardized the relationship, she, too, would have sought professional help and extricated herself from the depths of despair, but this is only guesswork. More germane to fallout mates are the signals both depressed partners sent out along the way.

First came "I love you/I love you not," accompanied or soon followed by "I want/I do not want to be married." With these came assignment of all blame to the non-depressed partner. The paths began to diverge when Penny's spouse agreed to marriage counseling and Sam's rejected any discussion of their problems. While the counseling per se failed to help, it may have led Penny's husband to see that the problem had two faces, thus sowing seeds of doubt that germinated along the way and gained strength from Penny's insistence on communicating her feelings and point of view. The flourishing of self-doubt on his part, nurtured by his past serious episode of depression, led him eventually to see a psychiatrist and then, further down the line, a psychotherapist.

Drawing the conclusion that Sam somehow failed in his role as spouse of a depressed mate is the wrong one; the more likely explanation is that his wife's depression took them both by surprise. Unaware of its presence and destructive potential, neither was prepared for the fault lines in communication and trust that must have preceded the full force of its eruption. When it came, Sam had little to build on other than love for his wife and his hope that the toxicity of the marital relationship would abate before his tolerance for stress and misery gave out. In the end, his wife's depression triumphed and left great losses in its wake.

Foresight is a lot more useful than hindsight. Choosing between staying and leaving might have been easier if Sam had asked his wife some tough questions:

- Will you acknowledge depression as a possible cause of our problems?

- Can you admit to inner turmoil and doubt?

- Will you, under well-defined circumstances, agree to periodic discussion of the issues between us?

- Will you try to understand and abide by my needs list, and will you give me one of your own?

- Do you really want to start divorce proceedings, or are you perhaps hoping that I will, and that that will relieve you of the onus of "quitting"?

- Do you want a trial separation? If yes, for what purposes and for how long?

- Will you agree to consult a psychiatrist and to take medication if prescribed?

- Will you pledge to continue the medication for at least six months?

- Will you start psychotherapy?

- Will you agree to work on our problem together?

Answer by answer, an outline of the shape of things to come emerges. Not every negative response predicts failure: To this day, Penny's husband (now on his second, and for him more effective, antidepressant) still refers to his depression as a sleep disorder. Other depressed mates dodge discussion of a mate's needs list, yet work to meet them nonetheless. But some negatives, especially if they are long-standing and show no sign of softening as time ticks by, are bad omens. One is the refusal to talk even when fallout partners follow the rules governing communication with the depressed. Another is refusal to see a psychiatrist, even when this is laid down as the condition for saving the relationship. Both augur poorly for a joint future.

Reading signals as positive or negative is, in the absence of a crystal ball, the best predictor of what the end of the story will be. Oldtimers who provide updates on their ex-partners indicate that a combination of severe depression and refusal to seek help does not lead to miraculous turnarounds in the absence of spousal pressure, nor are there any tales of extramarital affairs that have endured. The good news appears limited to workable arrangements vis-à-vis children. Phil, who is still using humor to help him cope, says that his ex-wife's anger at life in general and at him in particular is alive and well. In her usual cranky voice, she called him recently to say she was furious because she could not remember the plumber's name; "I totally accept responsibility," he wrote, "because even though she had never told me his name, I should have known it." She was mad at the bank because the machine ate her card; "I fully accept blame for that, too." In fact, he continued, after pondering long and hard over why everything was always his fault, he had come to a logical conclusion: "It's because I have blue eyes, my blood group is 'O,' and my belly button doesn't stick out."

Windswept's bipolar husband has become a recluse and lives alone in a wood-bound cottage, seeing only his parents and his son and daughter-in-law, who visit him once a month. Just Me says her ex-husband is still taking his antidepressants, together with large amounts of alcohol, but hasn't seen his psychiatrist in ages and has discontinued psychotherapy. When he calls Just Me, it is to say he still wishes they could have worked things out but understands why this is not possible. Prism's husband is miserable but unrelenting: no medication, no therapy, no effort to heal the breach. She suspects he might actually be happier in his own way. "I don't think he can handle the emotional responsibility of a marriage anymore," she observed. "I think he does best when his life is simple, with few moving parts, so to speak."

There is no way to ascertain the success and failure rate of all relationships touched by depression. Surely many of them do survive and prosper, but to be fore-warned is to be forearmed.

## THE DEPRESSIVE VERSION OF CHINESE WATER TORTURE

For the majority of fallouts, the line between staying and leaving is fuzzy. They toy with crossing it but are restrained by hope, guilt, and all the other considera-tions—finances, the welfare of children, fear of living alone—that attend any divorce or breakup with a long his-tory. Some depressed partners do pack up and go, but most doggedly elude taking action, instead maneuvering themselves into a position at dead center and then push-ing the envelope until their mates are finally driven to make the decision for them. This plays out as a repetitive cycle akin to Chinese water torture: a patch of particularly wretched behavior on the depressive's part, breakup threats from the fallout mate, followed by behavior that looks like an honest attempt to reform, and then by back-sliding and more fallout cries of pain. Every time divorce is mentioned, depressed mates have a comeback to dodge blame for ending the relationship: "Oh well"—(deep sigh)—"if that's what you want," "How can I help when you're always so negative?" or "If you only knew how much pain I'm in." These comments, which contain a grain of truth, are intended to raise their partners' hopes and shake their resolve. Fueling them is the perverse need of the depressed to confirm their belief that they are indeed unloved, and that should the relationship come to an end, it will not be their fault.

Moving forthrightly toward divorce frightens depression sufferers. The grass over there may look greener to them, but thanks to their emotional fragility and conflicting desires, sitting on the fence seems safer. Manipulation allows them to stay there, and they count on partners to opt for even a brief ray of hope. This explains why depressed partners talk about but shrink from initiating divorce proceedings, a tactic exemplified by Aurora's husband, who is tilting with depression for the third time in seven years yet still refusing professional help. When Aurora gave up attempting to communicate with him, principally to avoid being shouted at and bullied, her husband said he couldn't stay married to someone who refused to talk to him. Instead of calling his lawyer, he instructed her to find a lawyer of her own so she could be sure of her rights, and the next day claimed he did not want to be divorced. Other fallout mates have reported almost identical scenes with an added fillip: In the relative calm that follows the bomb, they are treated to the hugs and caresses they had longed for in earlier fallout stages.

Non-depressed partners, worn down and emotionally wrung out, feel like pawns on a chessboard. Checkmated at every turn, they dither and simmer resentfully, and their emotional stress balloons. One option is to postpone a final decision and suggest a temporary separation.

## THE PROS AND CONS OF A TEMPORARY SEPARATION

The most evident benefit of a trial separation is that it offers both partners time to reflect on the future in an atmosphere of relative calm. Freed from abrasive interaction on a daily basis, fallout partners are able to gain a measure of objectivity and observe their reactions to living apart. Other potential benefits depend on the circumstances under which the separation has been negotiated: Which partner proposed the separation? Was it preceded by an ultimatum that laid out the conditions under which reconciliation was possible? Were time limits imposed?

The Message Board experience suggests that when depressed mates decide to leave against their partners' wishes, they are unlikely to return. The reason is rooted in the depressive psyche and its bleak view of the future. Guy's wife, recently prescribed a second antidepressant when the first failed to work, insisted on discussing the terms of a divorce because she "knew" the new drug wouldn't work any better than the old one, and so nothing had changed. Guy's reasoning was that they should wait a few months to see if the new medication helped, but soon after, checking the contents of the pill bottle, he discovered that his wife had been skimping or skipping her daily dose. Confronted with this sabotage, she asserted that Guy would emerge happier than she because she would be both unhappy and alone. Turning the screw, she predicted that, although she didn't know now what she wanted, she would regret her decision later. "My wife actually said that even so, she would be too damn stubborn to ask for forgiveness. That makes me feel as though I am the one in denial," he added, "that I am just dragging this out because I don't want to let her go."

Trying to do battle with depression demons as implacable as these will result in a string of defeats, each one further draining your emotional reserves. Painful though it is, calling the battle a draw and putting down arms is sometimes wiser than continuing to fight. Even in this situation, a separation may be helpful, if only to smooth your transition to being single again.

Luckier fallout partners, who rightfully perceive the possibility of a mate's change of heart and mind, should not leave the outcome to chance. If you take the initiative rather than leaving it in depression's hands and lay down some governing rules, a temporary parting will gain you more than time. During the months apart, your mate will be forced to consider what life is like without you, and to decide whether or not that prospect is tolerable; choosing to squarely confront the damage done by the illness as a condition for reconciliation may seem a more than reasonable price to pay for regaining a partner's love. Rules might include a three-month moratorium on all divorce talk, only one phone call to you per week allowed, and your promise that if at the separation's end your partner still wants to part permanently, you will sit down and work out amicable arrangements. If your depressed mate balks at these stipulations, be firm and tell him or her that you've put up with their decisions, their whims, and their illness, and now it's your turn to make the rules. Point out that if it's so difficult to go for a few days without speaking to you, why are they asking for a divorce?

Fallout partners who suggest separation are subject to attacks of guilt, especially those who in their own mind see this step as a prelude to divorce rather than as a chance to reconsider a permanent split. Their desire to escape unhappiness is muddied by issues of fairness. Separation begins to look like heartless abandonment of a mate already disabled by depression, and they worry that it could lead to increasingly rash behavior, such as sliding into alcoholism or drug use, performing badly at work, or even threats of suicide. A wise therapist asked Board poster Katie, who could not summon the courage to decide on separation, to make a list of all the fears that bore on the decision, and virtually every one of them related to the same question: Is it fair to leave a depressed person? This wife feared taking away the few things that made her husband happy—the children, the house he helped renovate, the dogs; she feared for his credit rating and his bank account; she feared for his job.

When making a decision, be careful that guilt is not a decisive factor against separation or divorce. Katie's fears may well be justified, but in order for her to address them constructively, they must be shared by her depressed spouse. Wringing your hands on the sidelines will not change your mate's self-destructive behavior, nor will your guilt force him or her to reappraise the future. If guilt continues to plague you despite rigorous introspection, consider that it may arise from the fear that you have failed to make clear to your partner precisely why you wish to leave and what it would take for you to alter the decision. Viewed in this light, a separation preceded by the preparatory steps suggested above will relieve you of the suspicion that you are doling out what your mate "deserves" for having inflicted emotional pain and at the same time open the door to eventual reconciliation based on reform.

The ability of one or the other partner to physically quit home base depends on a bank account that accommodates renting other quarters, or on parents or friends willing to offer a temporary bed. In their absence, it is possible to achieve emotional distance by dividing the apartment or house in half and sharing the kitchen and bath according to a set schedule. Some Board posters have managed this reasonably well, but only if they have been able to structure an independent social life and put their own needs first. Spending time with people who love you just as you are, enjoying the kids without having to protect them from scenes, and doing what you like brings its own reward—the return of self-respect.

Whether the distance is physical or emotional, it grants an opportunity for introspection that has been lacking. Fallout mates with time to think may discover within themselves an unexpected strength and purpose that quiets their internal chaos. What they learn may be a welcome surprise. Often, their grieving for their mates is qualified by a sense of relief, as though the clamor of noise had suddenly ceased, allowing them the luxury of listening to themselves. In this quiet, the choice between obsessively trying to change a beloved's depressive behavior and accepting it at one's peril begins to look one-dimensional, as though the door to a wider world opens and life beckons again. The sense that life is controlled by the partner's illness gradually eases, leaving more room for choice. Anchored more surely by a rebounding self-esteem, they may come to the liberating realization that ultimately, the choice lies not with them but with their partners.

## A TROUBLING QUESTION

A Board newcomer posed a troubling question in the form of an analogy: Would you leave someone who had cancer? But the analogy is flawed. Cancer patients work hard to get well and refuse further treatment only if they know their illness is terminal and prefer release to more pain. The panoply of treatments for depression holds out the promise of success in most cases, and acceptance or rejection of medication and psychotherapy is a choice only the depression sufferer can make. While it is understandable for non-depressed mates to think they have somehow failed if treatment is refused, the guilt is not theirs to own. Those who suffer from depression are free to fight against it or to give in; no one can force a choice upon them.

    Another poster came up with a more accurate analogy. "I know what you are fighting to avoid," she wrote in response to another's post about his wife's recalcitrant attitude to medication. "It's like watching a locomotive barreling down the tracks, knowing that the bridge up ahead has been washed out. You wave your arms, you scream frantically, pleading with the engineer to stop, but the train hurtles forward." If the engineer won't remove his earplugs, there is little the fallout mate can do to avert the crash.

Some depression sufferers dig in their heels and refuse to help themselves, but sometimes it's the illness that digs in and refuses to go away. Everyone who lives with serious depression also lives with the fear that one day they will wake up and find that the latest, and perhaps the only untried, drug regime has stopped working. Treatment-resistant depression puts another face on the leave-or-stay dilemma and poses a special challenge for both the depressed and their partners. Rising to this challenge is not for the fainthearted. Those forced to battle with chronic depression draw courage from the knowledge that a partner is in the arena with them and are more willing to try yet another combination of drugs or ECT instead of laying down their arms. Their mates, even though subject to emotional bullying, flip-flopping, and complaints, must accept that these stem more from the obdurate nature of the illness than from an unwillingness to get better. Filling the multiple roles of caregiver, cheerleader, and anchor of hope while monitoring treatment progress and keeping the household routine as normal as possible demands both love and a high tolerance for stress.

The more elusive wellness is, the more likely the depressed are to let the illness win. Some sufferers caught in this downward spiral choose to end the battle by committing suicide. The loving and supportive parents of one such young man were told by their son's psychiatrist—a doctor with a deserved reputation for solving tough cases—to prepare for the eventuality of suicide, saying, "He has given up because all the options have failed. Sooner or later, he will find a way to end his life." The warning was given to absolve the parents of guilt for their son's death. When their son did find the means to kill himself, the physician's words were key to the grieving process; without them, they might never have found closure.

## AN SUNG'S STORY OF HOPE

For every depression tragedy, there is a story of hope. After reading the Board for a while, An Sung decided his experience could be helpful to others. His wife had been diagnosed with depression and sought help for it, but full recovery was long in coming and marked by repeated treatment failures. During what he described as one of her darkest periods, An Sung's wife began an extramarital affair with someone she met on the Internet and she and her husband separated for almost a year before reconciling. Once back together, An Sung took the precaution of educating himself about the illness so that he would be better prepared if his wife suffered a relapse; when this indeed happened a few months later, both knew what to do. This time, he reported, with the right medication, a supportive therapist, and a lot of love, she is emerging on the other side.

The flesh An Sung puts on these bare bones of a story is what makes his experience and the insights it brought him valuable to fellow fallouts. "I was very supportive in all the outward ways a spouse is supposed to be. As she lay on the sofa for days on end, I fed her, cleaned the house, ran our business, and took her to doctor and therapy appointments. I did everything but the most important thing: I didn't tell her that I loved her unconditionally, that I would stay with her through the worst that depression could offer, and that we would walk out together on the other side. To the contrary, I was resentful of all that I had to do. I was sorry for myself. I didn't understand the illness, or the hell she was going through. All I could see was that I had lost my lover, my best friend, and my business partner all at once. But the man she met on the Internet, who had no real investment in her happiness, told my wife all the things I had forgotten to say. That man treated her with all the romance that tells a woman that she is beautiful and desirable. Even during our separation, I never stopped loving her and came to understand that I bore some responsibility for her pushing me away."

This husband wasn't interested in solitary sainthood; he wanted a second chance for the marriage. He knew his wife's lover had found an easy mark, but An Sung says that wasn't the issue, nor was losing a year of his marriage. He managed to resist hurling recriminations when they reunited and chose instead to spend a lot of time talking about how they could work together to prevent anything coming between them again. There is no minimizing the hurt and suffering that fallout partners experience at the hands of their depressed mates. The road to regaining trust, An Sung admits, is booby-trapped with pain, but sooner or later everyone has to make a decision whether or not to take it.

## SECOND CHANCES

Second chances are predicated on hope and trust. When one is present but the other is profoundly shaken, fallout partners hesitate to move forward without a road map of the territory to come. Some, even though they may still love their mates, run out of both and hit Caps Lock on their computers to express thoughts such as "I WILL NEVER GO THROUGH THE DARKNESS AGAIN!" and "THEY SHOOT HORSES IN THIS MUCH PAIN." Denise refers to her separation, which ended in divorce when her husband's return led straight back to a replay of all the same unresolved issues, as "a necessary amputation." Many fallout partners who do offer a second chance encounter yawning traps, some of their own construction: They know unfettered communication is mandatory, yet shrink from the clashes it may bring; they hope for truth, yet anticipate lies and slippery gambits that will leave them open to more hurt and disappointment.

Trying to gauge the prospects for success without some dispassionate input is a lonely and usually unrewarding task, but seeking it from family and close friends has its own pitfalls. Friends, unless also burdened with a depressed mate, agitate for an immediate and permanent end to what they see as self-punishment. Parents automatically leap to defend an offspring's interests as they see them; their views may be colored by ideas about marriage and the welfare of their grandchildren that do not concur with yours, and their understanding of depression is often outdated. In-laws are weighted by the same considerations. None of these potential sources of comfort and advice know how radically your partner has changed, having seen only the Jekyll mask; your tales of outrageous behavior may sound exaggerated. Solicit their support, but don't expend your energy on converting the unconvertible. You need professional help.

## AN EXPERT'S SLANT ON THE PROBLEM

Fallout mates and their depressed partners wrestle endlessly for control by using an age-old tactic: blaming each other for all the relationship's problems. But "every individual," says psychiatrist and couples counselor John Jacobs, "is a member of a system. The worst marriages are those in which each spouse focuses only on the other, and the self is never seen as part of a system." The depressed look for someone to blame for the awful way they feel and assume that just because they are depressed, everything they do and say is correct and permissible. Although understandable, says Jacobs, this is "a very dangerous attitude for them to take. The depressed really aren't well enough to realize they're jeopardizing their marriage and must mend their ways to save it." Fallout partners, worn down by the recurrent, frustrating disappointments they experience, "eventually arrive at a moment when they can't take it anymore and go over the cliff. Once that happens, the problems become irreconcilable."

Dr. Jacobs lobbies hard for joint sessions because improving communication is an essential step, but even when the depressed partner refuses to attend, his couples perspective prevails. When he takes on the job of repairing a relationship frayed by depression, Jacobs is alert to the possibility that unaired, unresolved conflicts predating the illness have been accentuated by it. Fallout partners often express themselves indirectly, harping on small annoyances instead of stating their real complaints—sexual rebuff or lack of respect, for example—which in Jacobs's view probably troubled the relationship well before the illness arrived but have never been openly aired by either partner. He cautions that depressed partners are poor listeners and incapable of reading between the lines, and warns that they, like you, harbor resentment about these unresolved issues. Sorting old problems from new ones provides clues to the relationship's overall dynamic and opens the door to remedial measures that will hold the union together until the depressed partner's denial is overcome.

If you have no Dr. Jacobs to help you identify hidden trouble spots—which may actually have triggered your partner's depression and are now reinforcing it—you can explore them by creating a nonthreatening opportunity for your depressed partner to come out with what's really bothering him or her. A Jacobs script would read as follows: "Honey, I know you feel terrible. Please let me know what I can do to help you?" "Nothing." "I know that's not true; it's just that you don't want to tell me." Silence, due to apathy and the belief that he or she has already told a thousand times what's wrong, without any positive results. "Okay, so how about making a list of three things, in order of their importance, that I can do to improve your life and our marriage?" "This has nothing to do with my being depressed, but I wish you would . . ." With luck, the underground, preexisting issue that surfaces—"You criticize me in front of friends," "You're mean to my parents," "You get upset when I want sex and you don't"—will be something you can act on by changing your behavior. In the end a fallout spouse may say, "You know, honey, you're right about that, and I should have listened to you long ago. I'm going to make a real effort to stop doing that." Combined with a certain amount of empathy and sympathy, this strategy will reduce tension by putting more cards on the table; when denial of depression is overcome, the residual damage will be easier to repair.

Dr. Jacobs, a strong believer in medication, takes a proactive role because he knows what couples have to do to have a mutually gratifying relationship and sees no point in waiting for the depression to run its course. In the absence of a skilled and proactive counselor, balancing one's tolerance for depressed behavior with love for a spouse will help determine a choice between making and breaking the bond. You can construct the framework for a happy ending, but you can't force your partner to embrace it. You may offer your support and advice, but you can't mandate acceptance. And no matter how deep and true, your love doesn't guarantee that your mate will act as you wish. Once you have done everything in your power to preserve the relationship, have made your own views clear and listened to your partner's, your ability to dictate a joint future comes to an end.

## WHAT ABOUT THE CHILDREN?

Worries about children cast a giant shadow on any decision about divorce. One wife's post described a Sunday free of bickering until the couple's two young children put on a play at dinnertime that proved "too chaotic" for their depressed dad, who stamped out of the room midway to a chorus of shrieks and tears of disappointment. "Little by little, my expectations of what is 'normal' family interaction are becoming distorted," wrote Stephanie. "I could bear it if my husband's behavior affected only me, but I have a sense of futility about my future and the children's."

The torrent of replies confirmed the creeping disarray brought on by a parent's depression and its negative impact on kids: bad dreams, temperamental outbursts, and a breakdown of communication with their depressed parent are common. Although at times Stephanie's husband reverts to his old self, the kids now use their mother as an intermediary instead of addressing him directly, their way of coping with his emotional unavailability. Peter's son does the same, and every time Peter urges the boy to speak directly to his mother, it feels like "sending the poor kid into the lion's den." "I don't know how much longer I can keep lighting candles to protect my daughter from her father's depression," wrote another. "I feel we are all trapped in its darkness."

A parent's depression pulls children into its sticky web. Of all the illnesses a parent can have, chronic depression is the one most likely to disturb a child's emotional base. "Depression causes a huge disruption in nurturing relationships, even more so than schizophrenia or bipolar disorder," says Dr. Peter Jensen, director of Columbia University's Center for the Advancement of Children's Mental Health. "If a parent is prone to psychotic episodes, offspring, especially older ones, can separate what's taking place from reality and can say to themselves, 'Mom (or Dad) checked out today,'" Jensen explains, "but if a parent is constantly withdrawn, or critical, or unsupportive, because they're struggling with their own feelings, it feels like the real McCoy to kids." Instead of knowing they are cherished and feeling protected, these children come to see their position in the family as precarious, dependent on pleasing or appeasing the depressed parent, or on creating attention-getting scenes in hopes of some limelight and comforting. Soon the self-protective coping styles adopted at home spill over into their relations with peers and with authority figures at school. Unless the non-depressed parent takes preventative steps, they will become ingrained and endure, even if the children are no longer directly exposed to depression.

Experts in the domains of psychiatry, psychology, and child development have been studying depressed parents and their children for three decades. The behaviors and underlying feelings they have identified in these offspring are age-related. Infants of a depressed mother are less likely to thrive physically and are less responsive and secure in their attachment to their parent. Other consequences show up as behavioral and learning problems among toddlers and school-age kids. In adolescents, they play out as poor grades and in such social shortcomings as low self-esteem, trouble making friends and handling authority, lack of emotional equilibrium, and drug and alcohol abuse. Some of these develop over time, but others manifest themselves immediately. When Harvard researchers asked a group of young mothers to pretend for a few minutes that they were depressed by keeping their face still and unresponsive, the effect on their babies was dramatic. Almost at once the infants detected the change in their mothers and tried to get their attention. When the infants failed to get any reaction from their mothers, they looked away, then tried again, and repeated this cycle several times before finally giving up and slumping dispiritedly, comforting themselves as best they could.

The research focuses on maternal depression because mothers are assumed to be the primary caregivers, but common sense dictates that a father's illness will cause many of the same problems. All depressed parents tend to be negative, critical, quick to anger, and emotionally detached, and these impede a close and loving relationship. When researchers took a look at children who felt close to their dads growing up, they found that they were twice as likely as those who did not to enter college and find stable employment after high school, 75 percent less likely to have a teen birth, 80 percent less likely to spend time in jail, and half as likely to experience multiple symptoms of depression.

Dr. Jensen suggests protective strategies that depend on the child's age and on whether or not the depressed parent acknowledges having the illness. Very young children need a lot of shielding, but as the child grows older, says Jensen, "the well parent can help him or her understand that what's taking place isn't their fault, that mom or dad is just having a bad spell." Because this may seem like undercutting the other's parenting role, he suggests saying something like, "You *can* expect more from Mom, but this isn't the time to get it because she isn't feeling well right now."

A special, particularly close relationship often develops between the well parent and the child. "When the depressed parent tries to reassume his or her parenting role, they may feel out of it and rejected," Jensen says, unless the well parent is willing to pull back and allow the other to reassume his or her previous parenting role. "By then the child may have grown very resentful of the depressed parent. If this happens, the well parent needs to say, 'You're not being fair to Dad. He was having a tough time, and he's really trying. If you were having a tough time, you'd want some help, too, so you have to cut him some slack.' By the way," Jensen adds, "I've seen a lot of wonderful examples of fathers who have risen to the challenge of a new, more active nurturing role."

Working out a parenting partnership is extremely problematic in the presence of obdurate denial of depression. "When a depressed parent lacks any insight into the illness, he or she looks outside instead of inside for its reasons. That's dynamite," says Jensen, who despite years of working with such parents has yet to find any reliable formula for overcoming denial. "Direct exposure to chronic, overt conflict between parents is more harmful to kids than the death of a parent. If the depressed parent starts an argument, and the other says, 'I refuse to discuss that,' that's a conflict." A better course—in addition to presetting a boundary—is to ask him or her to save it for later, or to just refuse to engage and change the subject. But perhaps the best curb of all is to share with your depressed partner what you now know about the impact of depression on kids.

## LOOKING FOR CLOSURE

When everything has failed to heal the breach, fallout partners discover that the task of ending a relationship with a depressed mate has more than its share of the residual emotional and practical problems that follow any divorce. The break is rarely clean. It is sullied by the recurring pattern of even well-medicated depressions. Depressed partners may well approach their future in the same dispirited manner as they have their immediate past, leading one fallout partner to observe that the considerate, empathetic, honorable person she had married was handling the end of their union as though it were an eighth-grade romance. In trivializing the reasons for the breakup as "too much 'stuff' to handle," yet in the next breath eloquently admitting to their own unworthiness, the depressed twist the knife and reinforce the incipient guilt most fallout spouses harbor. Achieving closure, hard though it may be, is a prerequisite to moving on, and the burden of attaining it lies with the non-depressed.

No one on the Message Board had been able to resolve this satisfactorily until Jay held a funeral for his marriage. One glorious fall day, Jay rode his bike to the crest of a nearby hill, a mile above the inn where he and his wife, Nell, had celebrated their match six years earlier. He brought with him his wedding ring; his favorite photograph of Nell; a cheap pen she had given him years before their marriage when, as a teenager, he had helped her with a calculus assignment, and which he had used to write all his love notes to her, and every anniversary and birthday card; and a small notepad. Jay found a spot under a giant evergreen, then sat and thought, not about the bad times, but about all the good times they had shared. Then he wrote one last note to his wife: "I love you, Nell, and I always will." He put the note, together with his mementos, into a plastic bag and buried it there, then rode home again to greet the rest of his life.

One poster, moved by Jay's ritual burial, thought herself incapable of such an equally graceful closure because she had held on for too long and was too full of anger and thoughts of vengeance. Jay's accomplishment was his realization that he could not rescue his wife from her black hole without her help, and so he let her go and wished her well. By attaining closure, he held on to the good things they had shared together and shed his bitterness.

Stubborn love for their pre-depression mates is characteristic of the Message Board fallout partners. Were they able to give it up easily, their anger would be more amenable to control, its roots less tenacious and closer to the surface. But anger is not biodegradable. It can linger on and poison the good memories. While anger has its place in the grieving process, fallouts who use it to sever the bond may find they have only deepened their own bitterness, discoloring the future as well as the past.

Life beyond depression fallout, with your well-medicated partner or on your own, can be joyful, as you will discover in the final chapter.

# 9

# Life Beyond
# Depression Fallout

Is there life beyond depression fallout?" queried one spouse on the day her divorce became final. The answers, as varied as the posters who provide them, are positive; sooner or later, the sun breaks through the clouds. Problems that appeared insoluble—loneliness, bitterness, distrust, atomized self-esteem, residual guilt—slip into the past, and a future begins writing its story. Some posters are sharing the future with their partners, some with new ones, and others with their children or on their own. All who have made a definitive decision are fallout-free.

Fallout-free is not synonymous with problem-free, any more than one sunny day invariably predicts that another will follow. Problems have solutions; finding a workable one requires courage and belief in one's strength and purpose. Partners who opt to stay with their depressed mates must juggle their own emotional well-being and security with depression's demands; this equation is possible. The issue for others is the quality of the post-breakup relationship, of essential importance to those who have children; for them, the challenge is summarized in the oft-raised question "Is it possible, or wise, to remain friends with your ex-depressed partner?" The answer is usually yes. Reports from posters who have rediscovered love with a new partner challenge those still in stage five who insist, "Nothing can replace the lonely feeling in my heart."

## STAYING PUT

Your real partner, the one with whom you fell in love, has stepped out of the shadows with medication's help. This is indeed cause for rejoicing, but he or she has brought some baggage with them. They are wiser than before and their values are back in order, but they also carry the memory of their depression and the fear that it will return. Make room in your life together for both. The structure of a mutually gratifying relationship rests not just on shared love, but also on good communication and understanding of each other's needs. Unexpressed love, unanswered questions, and buried feelings will destabilize the heart's foundations, as will shards of old resentments and anger. Partners must learn from the past and then bury it. The sole permissible, indeed unavoidable, remnant from troubled times is the illness. Even when well controlled by antidepressants, the depression will continue to make its presence known through its waxing and waning lifestyle and in acquired habits of negative thinking.

Every depressed partner who has contributed to the Message Board has emphasized the need for constant reassurance from their mate that they are loved and will not be abandoned. Should you consider that finding ways to say "I love you" at breakfast, lunch, and dinner is gilding the lily, remember your fallout feelings when your "Do you love me?" was answered with "Well, I'm still here, aren't I?" This is the time for some excess; no successful relationship has foundered on exorbitant declarations of cherishment.

You now know the inner workings of the depressed mind. Do not expect your mate to change dramatically overnight, or in some cases, even after months or years. Depression settles on the personality like city grime on a windowpane, so expect even your well-medicated mate to have bouts of blurred vision and, if the illness has been around for a time, some permanent blind spots. "I am learning to recognize the symptoms that precede a fight or a crash and can now avoid much of my reactive behavior," a depressed partner explained to the Message Board. "My problem is that I learned this too late, after my wife fell out of love with me." The more your depressed partner can see his or her behavior and misperceptions as products of an illness, the clearer their perception of how much you are doing for them will become. While depression sufferers do learn how to monitor the course of their illness—some call it "owning their depression"—and to moderate their reactions to it, they will benefit from your impartial perspective. Non-depressed mates can learn that a sleepless night will probably be followed by a touchy day, for instance, or a small disappointment by disproportionate brooding and edginess. These are times to tread cautiously and to offer distractions.

Non-depressed mates should also bear in mind that a depression that has dug in for a long stay does not keep to a level course. At times it will hide out for so long that sufferers believe they are free of it at last and cautiously lower the dose of their antidepressant or stop taking it. Energy and contentment levels may remain elevated for months, and the only lurking problems with which the sufferer and you must contend are the bad habits acquired while the illness was in the ascendant: a tendency to anticipate disaster when none is brewing, a jaundiced view of one's abilities, or suspicions of unworthiness. And then, without reason or warning, the depression comes out of hibernation and starts plodding upward, slowly at first and then gathering speed, until the protective barrier of medication gives way. Major waxing or waning may occur every six or nine months (no one can predict the timing), while minor ups and downs can occur overnight. Every time a down comes, the "well" depressed worry that their medication has failed for good, and that the psychiatrist will have nothing else to offer. In all such matters, the partnership approach (and that includes psychiatrist and psychotherapist) will act as a safety net.

Depression fallout, like the illness, needs time to heal. When the fabric of a relationship has been torn, allowing distrust and resentment to enter, gaping rents will remain. Mending them is a two-person task, but while frank communication between partners is of critical importance, non-depressed mates, like their partners, must monitor themselves for signs of reactive habits formed during the bad old days. If you continue to interpret every withdrawal on your mate's part as lack of affection, and every half-truth as a deliberate lie, rebuilding mutual trust will be a long haul. A still-married wife had complained bitterly last year that her husband habitually criticized her appearance and social inadequacy before a dinner party and then called on the guests to join him in a toast to his beautiful, gracious wife. When asked recently for an update, she seemed surprised and answered that he rarely did that anymore. Why? "I don't know," she said. "Maybe he eventually got the message that it upset me, or maybe I just stopped making a big deal about it." The correct answer is not important; what counts is that the wife has let go of the past, and triggers that activated acute distress back then are rusty now. When her husband's depression gathers force, she applies a dash of Teflon and distracts herself by spending more time with friends. Instead of trying to coax her husband into a country weekend with friends, she goes by herself and has a good time.

Depression has a long memory, and the social withdrawal mandated by the illness causes many depression sufferers to shrink from engagement with others despite an improved view of the world. Reentry is best achieved when partners devote themselves first to mending the family bond. When Sally separated from her depressed husband, it shocked him into a visit to a psychiatrist and soon to a psychotherapist as well. Six months after his acceptance of a diagnosis of depression, Sally and their two-year-old have moved back home, and the family is learning how to enjoy life together. "No-pressure situations seem to work best for us. Some of the things we have done together: rented a movie and eaten Japanese takeout, taken the baby to the zoo, went tubing down the river, had a barbeque for the three of us, cooked omelets together, danced with our daughter to a Madonna video. Just simple little everyday things remind us both why we chose to be together in the first place."

## HAVING DOUBTS

In the early days of reconciliation, non-depressed mates may find it difficult to accept the reformed partner as the person with whom they fell in love. Your past history has already included two distinct people, one gentle and loving, the other mean as hell, so just exactly *who* is this partner number three? The answer is, the best one of all. Depression is a trial by fire, and those who have gone through it are often far more insightful, and far more grateful and devoted, mates than when you met them. They value happiness and security above all else and wish to share them with you.

Amy and her husband are back together, yet "now that he's saying all the right things, I'm having doubts!" Heart-broken by the pain he was going through, Amy had longed for him to come back home, "but I have been hurt so much. I want to have it made up to me, I want hearts and flowers and kisses." She admits that her husband has never been a hearts-and-flowers man, and although passionate in bed, he rations his kisses at other times. "Any suggestions?" "I understand so well," replied a husband, who offered his pre-scription. "When I'm doubting, I let myself have doubts and write them in my journal. Often, I'm as up and down about our relationship as my wife is with her depression. I try not to draw any conclusions from her behavior when I'm at either extreme. You're allowed to take things as slowly as you need to feel comfortable and confident."

Gwen took a more stoic stance about her misgivings, which she believes are normal and part of any reunion scenario. "There's a natural built-in resentment. Here we fallout partners have been wanting to work on the relationship all along, and that wasn't worth squat to our depressed mates, but when *they* finally want to work on it, it's supposed to be confetti and parades all around." Gwen's solution was to clench her teeth and try her best despite negative feelings, because she had worked hard for this moment and wasn't going to let it turn sour. "And sure enough," she wrote, "once things really started solidifying, I did find myself feeling genuinely happy about it. I started being able to use the cynicism acquired during bad times as backbone to improve the relationship, and I began looking at my as yet unrealized expectations to find out what new things I could put into our life together that would fulfill my desires."

Patrick takes a long and generally hopeful view of life with his depressed wife that is buttressed by attentiveness to his own needs. After a decade of proximity to his wife's illness, he had thought of himself as a half-healthy man who had lost the capacity for happiness. When he realized that he had grazed bottom and could no longer withstand the avalanche of her despair, Patrick's first reaction was relief and "some small satisfaction that I was off the hook, free to stop trying to understand or help my wife." But that didn't last. Patrick decided to "take care of my own garden, bring light and sunshine back into my own life." This has, he says, renewed both his desire and his capacity to help his wife, "whom I have never ceased to hold very dear indeed, and who even in her blackest periods is a fine and loving mother to our wonderful children."

Accept that most non-depressed partners have doubts and that depressed mates have them, too, but don't embrace them so tightly that there is no room for hope. If your mate is bipolar you have already earned an advanced degree in doubting. Hang on to what you have learned about your partner's mercurial behavior and be aware that he or she probably finds their current medicated life a hard step down from the headiness of high altitudes. Even psychosis and hospitalization in the past cannot be counted on to repress memories of unbridled freedom. Your manic-depressive mate is surely wondering, "What if you only like me when I'm my crazy, entertaining self? What if you find me boring now?" The answer to give before the question is asked is that your love isn't going to disappear because of ups and downs. Say that you place great value on the effort to stay steady, and that you are basking in the comforts of regained intimacy.

The shaken confidence and low self-esteem that make chronic depressives prone to negativity also make them extremely responsive to support, encouragement, and praise. Should your supply of these be inadequate to the task, now is the correct time to try couples counseling. As the Message Board experience bears out, however, seeking this help when one partner is deeply depressed can actually widen the rift by eliciting honest but unwelcome assessments such as "I don't know if I want to stay married." But now that you know their origin, and your partner is out of denial and on medication, a skilled couples counselor can smooth the way to mutual understanding. Previously the issue was "Why can't my partner get it?" The issue that needs attention now is "How can we help each other and iron the wrinkles out of our relationship?" Counseling will improve the quality of communication between you and your partner and will mediate missteps until each of you can accurately hear and accept what the other is saying, instead of inferring meaning based on past experience.

## EXCHANGING VIEWS THROUGH THE MESSAGE BOARD

A couple having a rough time of it inadvertently turned the Message Board into a couples counselor when a medicated but still depressed partner, Melody, used her own experience to clarify depressive thinking and behavior for some puzzled fallout posters. The problem, said Melody, is her inability to explain to her longtime boyfriend how she really feels about their three-year relationship and why she keeps pulling away from him. The evening before posting on the Board, Melody had promised her beloved that she would try to communicate better and that she would send him a long explanatory E-mail, "But today I am having such a bad day that I want to be left alone . . . he has called three times and left a message saying he's not trying anymore . . . I feel panic because I think he is giving up on me . . . I feel pressure . . . I don't call because we'll have an argument . . . and because I don't want to talk about me." Melody's post wound up with a list of her acknowledged faults: She pushes her boyfriend away, doesn't talk, won't meet, can't commit, feels guilty, believes he deserves better and that the relationship should end.

Within hours, sandwiched in between questions from posters who wanted to know what non-depressed partners should do in such situations, was a reply from Mac: "I am the guy Melody is talking about." Addressing himself in part to Melody and in part to the Board in general, Mac said he only wanted to give Melody the love she deserved and that he had thought her communication-dodging a game. He admits to ambivalence and frustration. "Everyone needs space, but that shouldn't mean shutting others out. Trust me, everyone, I have everything that Melody needs and I want to give it to her, but it frustrates me that she won't take it. Melody, I don't see this as me giving up on you, but as your depression giving up on us."

Instead of answering Mac directly, Melody chose to respond to another poster's queries. A fallout husband trapped in the same noncommunicatory bind with his depressed wife wanted to know where the line was between pushing when Melody needed help and pushing too far, and how Mac could support her when she wants to "just be alone." "He needs to push hard, but he also needs to understand that when I am acting that way it's because I'm at my lowest—I feel insecure, alone, and worthless, and want to hide from everybody, and mostly from myself. He needs to tell me he's not going to tolerate that behavior." Melody's answer to the second question was that Mac shouldn't back off when she says she wants to be "alone to deal with it myself. I can't deal with it alone, this I now know. When our minds tell us that we should keep everybody at a distance so they can't hurt us, that's the depression thinking. When we are pressured and feel like running, all part of the illness, please don't demand that we talk—instead, express your concern, reassure us, ask us if we are able to talk."

During the ensuing week, the couple, cheered on by other posters, used the Message Board to break the communication deadlock. They had tried to talk face-to-face, but Melody couldn't tell Mac clearly that she loved him. Freaked out, she had skipped her therapy appointment. "I want you to know that I do love you and I feel you in my heart," she wrote to Mac on the Message Board, "but I don't love myself right now so it's hard to communicate to anyone else how I feel. I'm sorry for that, and sorry, too, that we didn't spend New Year's Eve together. Next year will be better, I promise." By January eighth, on the eve of Melody's departure on a business trip, their Message Board posts were paeans of mutual praise and love. "I believe you have many reasons to love yourself," wrote Mac. "Let me go through them for you:

- You have a great smile that makes me smile.

- You're very smart.

- You're responsible.

- You're understanding.

- You care for others.

- You give me advice when I most need it.

"There are many more," Mac added, "but I think you get the gist. Valentine's Day is coming soon, and you can bet on being mine. Travel safe. I love you, baby!" "I love you, too," Melody replied. "Thanks for posting on the Board. I know you're doing it to help me get better, but you're helping others as well. You're just so wonderful that way. This is short because I know you're going to call in five minutes and I want to hear your voice saying good night to me." "Way cool," observed a poster; "All I will say is, YOU TWO ROCK!" wrote another. One wonders if a couples counselor, even one experienced in the ways of depression, could have bridged the gap between these two lovers so successfully and so fast.

All the ingredients for clear communication between depressed and non-depressed partners are offered above; use them to keep your own relationship free of misunderstanding and lost opportunities. Own the depression jointly and tackle problems as a team. Learn to recognize when your mate needs space and silence, and when he or she needs you to listen and to offer affectionate gestures of support. In time the depression will become a blurry figure in the background of your relationship that knocks occasionally for attention but is no longer a major player.

## THRIVING OR SINKING ON YOUR OWN

Sustaining the impact of a partner's depression is a consuming task that forces one into negativity. Whether relieved of the burden by choice or of necessity, non-depressed partners must come to terms with their past history. Among those who have made the transition from being part of a couple to being single, the experiences of four posters now on their own demonstrate that adjusting to the new status is far easier for some than for others. While it may look as though each poster is in a different stage of the grieving process, their respective outlooks are already a good indication of what their immediate future holds in store.

## "What a Difference a Year Can Make"

Last year Tom was burning up the Message Board with rage and sorrow at having been dumped by his partner. During the holiday season, all he could do was cry. "I was a MESS! Wanted to die, couldn't work, couldn't envision a life without him. Now here I sit, happier than I've ever been." Tom is more than happy; he's writing a novel (not about depression) and has received encouraging feedback from friends in the publishing world. He has a new job, working full-time as a crisis social worker and helping people who are going through rough times in their lives, "just like I went through. I'm amazed at how things turned around for me. Keep a stiff upper lip, seek therapy, and keep plugging along. Eventually you'll get your life back."

Tom's new lease on life did not drop like manna from heaven; in truth, he turned things around by coming to grips with loss and then filling the hole left by his partner with new interests and accomplishments. One source of his effervescent cheer may be his new job; it's a reliable truism that in helping others, you also help yourself. Tom's work is paid, but being a volunteer accomplishes the same goal: enhancement of self-esteem. From a practical point of view, both paid and volunteer work put you on a schedule and create responsibilities that must be met, no matter how down and lonely you may feel; working in a crisis center, a hospital, or a soup kitchen will place you among people who are far worse off, and attending to their problems will, at least temporarily, help you forget your own.

Loneliness feeds on itself. Waking up to a schedule free of engagements may at first be a welcome change, but it runs the risk of becoming a constant reminder that now you really are entirely on your own. Get out your address book and call those friends you had stopped seeing. Reread the chapter on putting your own needs first and put the suggestions into practice. Expand your horizons. Take charge of your single life and make it work for you.

### "My Husband Left Me a Year Ago and My Thoughts Are Only of Him"

A poster once observed that it is sometimes necessary to issue oneself a DNR order: Do not resuscitate this relationship. Posters like Windswept can lose their way in mourning and confuse enduring anger with enduring love. When recently asked by a friend (or perhaps her therapist) if she was better off without her former husband—a bipolar sufferer who put her through hell and continues to strike from a distance—Windswept searched her soul and found she was more unhappy than before he left, "because I still love this man and miss him very much. I am feeling just as raw and hurt as a year ago."

It is not possible to toss thirty years of marriage on the garbage heap without immense grief and internal struggle.

A period of resentment and anger is justified, and a crisp anger may help to cut the bond. Yet Windswept went on to say, "I hate how this man's mental illness tore the family apart and spewed the innocent into Nowhere Land. He, however, is still secure in his bipolar disorder, still behaving the same way, only now he has no family to worry about." Windswept's unhappiness is a formidable problem to resolve; she has had to grieve, relocate, change her lifestyle, go to a therapist and to a doctor, take medications, and generally start her life all over again, all because of her husband. "I didn't ask to be made exhausted and depressed, and I resent having to seek out all this help in putting my life back together when I had a life before."

Everyone on the Message Board loves Windswept. We have all followed the heartbreaking story of a marriage destroyed by manic depression as though we were sitting next to her on the roller coaster of despair. When she used her amateur expertise in psychiatric illness to secure a part-time teaching job, her triumph was ours. When unrelenting stress and sorrow damaged her physical health as well as her psyche, we went with her to the hospital and held her hand. When she posted the above message, many rushed to respond with empathetic advice; among them was Ginger, who included with her sympathy an essay on the meaning of the word *love*.

There is love, the feeling, "which can be made up of lots of different stuff: attraction, shared history, bonding at a deep level that's hard to shake because it happens at a very primal place in our brains." Then there's love, the verb, which is what really counts: "It's loving actions and loving deeds. A marriage requires that two people give of themselves on a regular basis. If there's a long absence of loving actions coming from one partner, your husband, there isn't much of a marriage, is there?" The all-important insight offered by Ginger is that Windswept's feelings may be lying to her, that although her heart knows many things, it isn't "all wise," and that major life decisions require agreement between the heart and head. "Your primal brain tells you that you were happier with your husband. That's the bonding thing, coming from the more ancient part of your brain, whereas the cortex, the part of the brain that we 'grew' over the millennia and that separates us from the reptiles, can tell us when we're acting in primitive ways and helps us to act like thinking humans instead."

For Windswept and others who share her dilemma, taking a cool look at the evidence will bring the line between the past and the present into sharper focus. Partners who once were happy lived with a kind and caring mate; the arrival of unhappiness coincided with the mate's transformation into a mean, unloving person. Living with a negative, depressed, thoughtless person on whom you cannot count to return your love, or to be there when needed, has nothing to do with love. Q.E.D.: Windswept is no longer in love with her ex-husband, but she believes she is.

So what must Windswept do? Ginger's suggestion is to be "a better friend to yourself, the kind of friend that you need now, one that spurs you on to become the best you can be, helps you find the happiness within, and does the things that make your life meaningful and positive." The way to achieve that is to take one step at a time. Wake up every morning and make a list of three things for which you are grateful. Windswept's first list might be: (1) My son and daughter-in-law live nearby; (2) They love me and care about my happiness; (3) My depression (what caused it doesn't matter) is in control. The next morning she will find three more reasons to count her blessings; perhaps one is only that it is a beautiful day, or that a friend has invited her to lunch, or that she laughed while watching television. Acquire the habit, and the reasons will multiply like rabbits.

## "I've Made the Break, but My Self-Esteem Is Still in Tatters"

Carrying blame for undeserved failure can become a habit. Long after the final parting, the fallout mantra may go on buzzing in one's ears, as though the ego's self-portrait had been permanently redrawn. Clare, author of the above quote, has internalized the mantra's message; like many in her shoes, she continues to magnify her faults and trivialize her attributes, just as her ex-husband did. A Message Board poster, after reading a long series of mea culpas by fallout wives and lovers struggling with their self-image, sent an unbiased evaluation that deserves a wider audience: "So many of you tend to beat yourselves up way too much! Each and every one of you comes across as wonderfully caring and supportive. I hate the damage that has been done to your self-esteem. There are so many men and women out there who would truly love and appreciate someone like you."

Even though friends and family play the role of Greek chorus, assuring you that you are fault-free and that you will

make it on your own, you may need the help of a psychotherapist to put you back in touch with reality. Phil
summed up the therapeutic goal in his reply to Clare. "I, too,
have been where you are," he wrote, "but I'm beginning to
see the light up ahead. At first, I saw success as repairing the
damaged relationship. Now it's clear that success is being
happy and comfortable with where you ultimately arrive."
Think of the old partnership as yesterday's news. There are
snippets of information that are helpful, among them an
appreciation of the strength you mustered to carry you
through the bad times, but discard the rest. You were neither
weak nor unsupportive, nor are you a failure; these false negatives have no place in your new life.

The soft spots in your ego need toughening. With a
therapist's help, you will regain faith in yourself and in
your ability to make good judgments. Keep the memories
of the good pre-depression times shared together; continue to be concerned for your former partner's welfare,
and to do what is possible to help the transition to life
without you. But not everything is possible; that's why you
are no longer together. Your task is to rescue your own
self-esteem, not theirs. They are adults and have all the
information necessary for change; you have done your
part, and the rest is up to them. Concentrate on liking
yourself and on planning a positive future.

## "My Life Is Still Surreal"

Some partners become stranded in a surreal limbo. They
know the relationship is over, the divorce papers are as

good as in the mail, but they cling to the hope that inadequate treatment of depression is the only explanation of their estranged mates' desire to divorce. The day after his soon-to-be ex-wife came around to pack up her belongings, Richard posted a long cry of pain. "I still have hope," he wrote, "although I don't know why. I'm a lovesick fool, and I know it. I fear so much, hurt so much, and it's not getting a hair better." Richard's wife, no longer wearing her wedding ring, had asked if she could keep the dog and chattily told him she had started playing hockey again and was taking cooking classes. "This was a cold-blooded person I was dealing with—antidepressants working just fine, I see, going to therapy, putting her life in order without me."

The Message Board post that initiated this book asked why, in *How You Can Survive When They're Depressed,* I had written that only "cured" depressed partners leave a relationship, the view of many psychiatrists and psychologists. The Board's evidence indeed runs counter to that thesis, but in some instances the experts' view holds true; Richard's wife is a case in point. Antidepressant medication is a far cry from psychoanalysis, but for some depression sufferers, antidepressants, too, can "reconstruct" the ego and by so doing, recast the user's perspective of the past and the people with whom it was shared. Reflecting on friends made back then, the well-medicated depressed person may wonder why they were chosen as intimates and what their attractions were.

Perhaps when his wife issued him "a wake-up call," she was, albeit clumsily, trying to wake Richard up with words in the same manner that her medication has jolted

her into a new reality. And perhaps it is true, as she sometimes tells him on the phone, that she still loves him, but
that he is too proximate a reminder of her three years in a
black depression and so is no longer welcome in her new
depression-free world. Instead of praying to God to help
him remember that his wife's behavior toward him is
"sick" and decrying the "lock on her heart" that "time and
luck" will allow him to find, it is time for Richard to realize
that good depression treatment has changed his wife and
that for her, the change is healthy.

The thoughtful replies to Richard's posts appear to
have succeeded where his wife failed. "I am at the point
where I need to learn all I can about *my* tendencies from
this relationship," he wrote a week later. "I will never
achieve happiness if I don't learn what I need to do for me.
I have no control over what happens now. That's heartbreaking, but also kind of liberating," and it's also insightful. Later still, Richard writes that he feels "it's possible
that the Emperor has no clothes," and wonders, "Who's
crazy here? I will get better," he concludes, using the
future tense for the first time.

"As you can see from my own posts," commented
Mike, "I'm confused as to whether I'm the depressed person from whom all the problems source, or the depressee,
as it were, who is on the receiving end of the grief. I have a
growing suspicion of my inclination to bundle up my own
glitches, load them onto the shoulders of another, and
then walk away smelling of roses." Inspecting oneself from
a distance can uncover previously unrecognized tendencies and weaknesses; one suspects that Richard is catch-

ing sight of some of his own. Mike's depressed-or-depressee query bears investigating for another reason, pointed out by one of the Board oldtimers: "I predict that a significant number of fallout partners will, like myself, at some stage develop depression." Should this happen, the limbo will become even more surreal.

## CHECKING YOURSELF FOR SIGNS OF DEPRESSION

Depression does not always arrive when expected. The effects of stress, like smoking, are cumulative. Partners who have survived an onslaught of slings and arrows without succumbing may disregard depression's signs when they appear during recovery from fallout. It is normal to feel sad and to be overwhelmed by the challenge of structuring a new life, but should these feelings turn into a constant sense of hopelessness and helplessness, review with care the list of depression's symptoms.

Living with a depressed mate provides a distinctive perspective on the illness, one associated with ugly personality changes and behavior damaging to others. Because this consequence of depression doesn't apply to you, and despite all you now know about depression denial, chances are that you will blame your current malaise on your present circumstances; when life is in order again, you assure yourself, it will disappear. But putting one's life back together is the epitome of a stressful endeavor. Remember the depression-symptom rule: If every day for two weeks you have one of the first two symptoms (a persistent sad, "empty," or anxious mood and loss of interest or pleasure in ordinary activities) plus four of the others on the list (decreased energy, sleep and eating disturbances, difficulty concentrating and making decisions, irritability, and excessive, uncontrollable crying are the most likely), you are depressed. Go see a doctor.

If the doctor does not agree that you're in need of medication, and if you don't at the moment feel up to disputing that opinion, give yourself two more weeks. Write down a few sentences every day describing how your symptoms are doing: Better? Worse? The same? Pay particular heed to the quality of your sleep; good sleep is essential to mental and physical health, and changes for the worse are early harbingers of depression. Sleeping pills and tranquilizers (and alcohol, too) may give you the semblance of relief, but they also serve to mask the real problem. What you need is honestly won, purposeful energy, and that may come only with the help of an antidepressant. Call the doctor again, and this time, insist on what you need.

## STAYING FRIENDS

Establishing a friendly footing with someone who has rejected your love, lied, and been emotionally abusive seems a worthless and indeed impossible pursuit. But whether or not friendship has a place in the aftermath of separation depends on more than personal choice. Some depressed mates recuse themselves from all contact or move away, but a surprising number cozily sidle up to the idea of their ex-partner as best friend before the ink on the divorce papers has dried. "My former husband thinks we're just really good friends now, and I resent that in light of everything we've been through," Amy writes. "There's a certain attraction to keeping that connection, but every time I really think about it, I'm just so angry at myself for even considering it." As one poster put it, becoming friends feels like accepting crumbs when the cake is gone. If there are no children to consider, time may make the decision for you.

Hate and anger are high maintenance emotions; discarding them deliberately is kinder to the psyche. A period of minimal contact with your former partner helps speed the severance process, but look forward, not backward, and don't rekindle your anger. Allow yourself to be sad. Crying is not a sign of weakness, and tears can be purging; one former husband put them on his daily agenda by spending his afternoon coffee break sitting alone in his car. "Who wants to be a 'real man,'" he asked, "if it means being emotionally void?" But sooner or later, non-depressed partners have to come out of hiding and settle on a communication mode that if not entirely friendly at least permits civility.

Beware of rescue missions. Your former mate has long relied on you as his or her emotional glue, and divorce isn't going to change that. If your ex-mate is now on an antidepressant and trying hard to go it alone, a helping hand is charitable. A call to see how they are doing, an offer to drop off the mail or to keep the golf clubs and fishing tackle in the garage until they are permanently settled are considerate gestures, and you will like yourself better, and feel less guilty, for having made them. Spare your former partner from chipper news briefs on how much you enjoy your freedom and be genuinely pleased if he or she has good news to report. But do not get involved in what Ginger calls "charity work," or rescue missions. You were a good friend to this man or woman for a long time, patient through their indecisiveness, loyal and committed to the relationship. You have done all that you could, and now it is up to them. Think of their medication, and of their therapist and psychiatrist, as having taken over your supportive role.

Be especially wary of a mate still in denial about his or her depression. These black belts in manipulation won't give up easily. They will play on your lingering love and pity as they have before, and the push-me-pull-me games will continue. A poster describing herself as "well detached" notes that she is nonetheless very susceptible to any act of kindness or affection on the part of her former husband. "I am motivated by my love and my heart; he operates in a calculating manner." Perhaps this is true, perhaps not; your voyages into your ex-partner's mind have come to an end. It is true that he or she is ill and unhappy, but you have already told them why, and what to do. If you wish to be close friends, you risk a replay of the past. Even in such hard-case situations, civility is more useful than scowls and arguments. Lives once closely knit together have threads that can never be clipped; friends and family in common, alimony and child support, even shared custody of pets demand continuing contact. Keep that contact as emotion-free as possible and steer clear of invitations to get together "for old times' sake" until your independence is firmly rooted.

## GOOD NEWS ABOUT CHILDREN FROM THE MESSAGE BOARD

The Board's sad stories about children are those written before divorce. The parenting instincts lost to depression resurface once the marriage is over, and even fallout exes with little reason to hope that their offspring will ever enjoy the love of two parents have good news to report. Depressed fathers and mothers, even if still in denial about their illness and the reason for the family breakup, rise to the parenting challenge because they love their kids. The prospect of losing them elbows self-absorption aside and reignites parental devotion.

Non-depressed parents who mistake this devotion for self-interest unwittingly deny children the chance to reacquaint themselves with a loving mother or father. Keep in mind Dr. Peter Jensen's dictum to make room for your former partner when you consider the welfare of your children. Separate your past history from the child's experience of your ex-spouse. Children love their parents. When love is withheld, they continue to long for it, and while they may hide the longing by appearing resentful and criticizing the depressed parent, the wish and the need for his or her love and presence in their life endure. Mothers with sole custody should encourage their former partner to spend time on his own with the child; sometimes this means helping to repair their bond by standing aside and not interfering as it strengthens. When your son or daughter returns from an excursion or a weekend with Dad, share the child's pleasure and do not show your resentment.

Katie has gone back to work and worries about how her school-age kids will fare. "I pray, meditate, and do positive visualizations that they will come out of this okay. It won't be easy with me working full-time, but I know that we will make this work to the best of our abilities," she wrote to Phil, remembering his concerns about his sons' welfare. "It goes without saying that the hardest part of my divorce is not living with my children," Phil answered, "but they know they can depend on me to be there for them, to give the unconditional love and nurturing they need without any negative vibes and feedback. Surely, in the end this is the best way forward to an emotionally healthy adulthood. Good luck with your new job, Katie. If you're happy and feeling independent because of it, that can only provide more good feelings for your kids to soak up." That is the best advice that any divorced parent could receive.

Peter's divorce from his depressed wife came after two years of rancorous discord, a poor template for amicable sharing of their children's time. She still blames her depression on Peter and wants to know nothing about his life. "As far as my ex-wife is concerned, she would be quite grateful if I simply disappeared totally and utterly from the face of the planet," he writes and then adds, "if it weren't for the kids." This exception to her other feelings is the one that matters, and she is far from the only depressed parent to make it. Brad, also a depressed parent, acknowledges the truth of his former wife's assertion that his illness, then unmedicated, was the ruin of their relationship. Now on antidepressants and making sense of his life, Brad

says the turnaround was inspired by his love for his daughter, "because she needed me. I am going to be the best
father my daughter can have." Give your depressed ex the
same opportunity.

An anonymous ex-husband gets the last word: "I must
step back from my depressed wife and let her spread her
wings in an effort to fly. I cannot any longer be her safety
net—that's reserved for the children now. And I will try to
find a new relationship with her, one as coparent and friend."

## AM I STILL CAPABLE OF LOVING?

Lingering demoralization and a poor self-image team up
with learned distrust to shake the faith of ex-fallout partners in their capacity to love and to accept it in return.
Numerous long threads on the Message Board speak to
this: "Are we born losers?" "Are we the kind of person
who always makes bad choices?" "Have I become like her
[or him]?" "How can I ever trust someone again?" Other
threads, posted months later, summarize the answers: "I
can hardly believe it, but I've met this great new person."
There is not only life but love beyond depression fallout.

Predictably, good news comes from those who have
already reported success in weaning themselves from their
former partners. The weaning process may include some
(non-depressive) zigzagging. A poster who thought hers
completed had been dating a "sane, sweet" man for five
months; believing herself immune to her former lover, she
accepted his invitation to have dinner and exchange news.
Two glasses of chardonnay later, Denise knew she still

missed him, and wondered if it were possible to break her connection to him. In a Board post headed "Major foolishness!" Denise requested verification that she was not nuts.

Women have a limitless capacity for discussing the difference between loving and being in love, and the Board's female contingent went into action. "Love vs. in love? Heart vs. head?" wrote one. "Don't jeopardize the new relationship for the sake of nostalgia. I think I've become addicted to the pain, but you have a choice. Don't miss the opportunity for happiness and children." Another poster suggested that Denise was missing the man she had wanted her ex-lover to be. "It's okay to still 'love' your ex and to be in love with someone else." By the end of the exchanges, Denise had tagged the evening with her former husband as an "I miss you and your life is going on without me" dinner, and on reflection agreed that her love for her new boyfriend is different and that she must stop comparing the two men.

Fifteen months later Denise was married, a first for the Message Board. Her announcement post offered thanks for help in getting her over the rough spots and for encouraging her "to focus on what was important in my life. Good things happen when you are with a healthy mate." Katie, a year after posting concerns about being a single working mother, has been seeing a new man for several months. "I think I'm finally over the fears and hesitance I experienced at first. It was difficult to get used to being with someone completely open and straightforward, and who is constantly supportive and a joy to be with. Initially I couldn't quite believe that he was as accepting of me as he

seemed to be, but I've come around and am very apprecia-
tive of it now!"

I am waiting for the announcement that two Board oldtimers have completed what began as an empathetic
cyber-friendship on the Message Board and set a date for
their marriage. What I suspect were countless E-mails, followed by even more long-distance phone calls—first
between themselves, and then with their respective children and parents—were in turn followed by cross-country
trips. Both these former fallouts continue to post encouragement and advice to newcomers, but they have not yet
gone public on the Board. We met a year ago, together
with a few other posters, to talk about what this book
should contain. The fruits of that discussion, together with
the collective wisdom contained in the tall towers of posts
I have printed out over the past three years and drawn on
as research, are now yours. Use them well, and whatever
you decide to do, have no regrets.

# APPENDIX

# A Guide to Internet Resources on Depressive Illness

NONPROFIT ORGANIZATIONS OFFERING INFORMATION,
EDUCATIONAL MATERIALS, NEWSLETTERS, AND LOCAL
SUPPORT GROUP ADDRESSES

American Foundation for Suicide Prevention
(888) 333-2377
www.afsp.org

Anxiety Disorders Association of America
(301) 231-9350
www.adaa.org

Depression and Related Affective Disorders Association
(DRADA)
(401) 955-4647
www.med.jhu.edu/drada

Mood Disorder Support Group of New York
(212) 533-6374
www.mdsg.org

This organization runs excellent weekly support groups for sufferers of depression and also for friends and family members. Click on "Depression in the News" for links to sites providing mental health news and information.

National Alliance for the Mentally Ill (NAMI)
(800) 950-6242
www.nami.org

Click on "Support" and then on "Local Affiliates" for addresses and phone numbers of local chapters.

National Alliance for Research on Schizophrenia and Depression (NARSAD)
(800) 829-0091
www.mhsource.com/narsad/html

National Depressive and Manic-Depressive Association (NDMDA)
(800) 826-3632
www.ndmda.org

Click on "Support Groups and Chapters" to access addresses of U.S. affiliates as well as a list of overseas groups.

National Foundation for Depressive Illness (NAFDI)
(800) 239-1265
www.depression.org

National Mental Health Association
(800) 969-6642
www.nmha.org

National Mental Illness Screening Project
(800) 573-4433 (Depression Screening)
www.nmisp.org

Each year a date in October is designated National Depression Screening Day; participating hospitals and clinics offer free screening for depression.

Postpartum Resource Center of New York
(631) 582-2174
www.postpartumny.org

Postpartum Support International (PSI)
(805) 967-7636
www.chss.iup.edu/postpartum


## GOVERNMENT ORGANIZATIONS

National Institute of Mental Health (NIMH)
www.nimh.nih.gov

This is the official Web site of the National Institute of Mental Health. In addition to providing information on depressive illness, this Web site allows you to read on-line the Surgeon General's *Report on Mental Health;* the supplement on *Mental Health Culture, Race, and Ethnicity;* the

Surgeon General's *Report on Children's Mental Health;* and the Surgeon General's *Report on Suicide Prevention.*

National Library of Medicine
www.ncbi.nlm.gov/pubmed

Offers abstracts of research on depressive illness published in professional journals.

## ADDITIONAL WEB SITES

Thousands of Web sites devoted to depressive illness can be located through search engines, of which www.google.com is one of the best, but not all Web sites provide accurate information. Those that follow are well established and reliable.

www.depressionfallout.com

Click on "Message Board" to access the cyber-support group on which *Depression Fallout: The Impact of Depression on Couples and What You Can Do to Preserve the Bond* is based.

www.lib.uiowa.edu/hardin/md/index.html

This Web site, maintained by the University of Iowa, has an exhaustive list of links to organizations and educational institutions throughout the world concerned with depressive illness.

www.mcmanweb.com

Maintained by John McManamy, who is bipolar, this is an excellent Web site to recommend to someone who suffers from depression and/or mania.

www.medscape.com

Click on "Register" to receive an on-line weekly newsletter about breaking news and research in psychiatry; specify that you are a "consumer" and your interest is "psychiatry."

www.mhsource.com

Click on "Disorders" under "Resources" for a list of psychiatric illnesses, most of which have links to "Ask the Expert: Consumer Questions," ranging from "The Best Antidepressant" to "Both Depressed." Click on "Depression" under "A–Z Disorders" to access the Depression Info Center; click on "Medical Information" to access a five-year archive of articles from *Psychiatry Times* listed by topic. Click on "Links" for sites related to depressive illness grouped by topic. Click on "Patient/Caregiver Support" for relevant articles.

www.psycom.net/depression.central.html

This Web site, maintained by psychiatrist Dr. Ivan K. Goldberg, provides exhaustive information on depressive illness. Click on "Psychiatrists Specializing in the Treatment of People with Mood Disorders" for a list of experts. Click on "Drug Treatment for People with Mood Disorders" and then on "Generic and Trade Names of Psychiatric Medications" for a list of all medications currently used in treating depressive illness.

www.rxlist.com

Type in the brand or generic name of any drug to access basic information for consumers on antidepressant medications. Click on "Advanced Search" for additional information such as dosage range, side effects, possible interactions with other medications, and a report on the drug's clinical trials.

# SELECTED
# BIBLIOGRAPHY

Jamison, Kay Redfield. *Night Falls Fast: Understanding Suicide*. New York: Alfred A. Knopf, 1999.

———. *Touched with Fire: Manic-Depressive Illness and the Artistic Temperament*. New York: Free Press, 1994.

———. *An Unquiet Mind: A Memoir of Moods and Madness*. New York: Alfred A. Knopf, 1995.

Kramer, Peter D. *Listening to Prozac: A Psychiatrist Explores Antidepressant Drugs and the Remaking of the Self*. New York: Viking, 1993.

———. *Should You Leave?* New York: Penguin Books, 1999.

Manning, Martha. *Undercurrents: A Therapist's Reckoning with Her Own Depression*. San Francisco: HarperCollins, 1994.

Martin, Paul. *The Healing Mind: The Vital Links Between Brain and Behavior, Immunity and Disease*. New York: St. Martin's Griffin, 1997.

The National Depressive and Manic-Depressive Association. *Restoring Intimacy: The Patient's Guide to Maintaining Relationships During Depression*. The National Depressive and Manic-Depressive Association, 1999.

O'Connor, Richard. *Undoing Depression: What Therapy Doesn't Teach You and Medication Can't Give You*. New York: Berkley Books, 1999.

Real, Terrence. *I Don't Want to Talk About It: Overcoming the Secret Legacy of Male Depression.* New York: Scribner, 1997.

Roan, Sharon L. *Postpartum Depression: Every Woman's Guide to Diagnosis, Treatment, and Prevention.* Holbrook, Mass.: Adams Media Corporation, 1997.

Sheffield, Anne. *How You Can Survive When They're Depressed: Living and Coping with Depression Fallout.* New York: Three Rivers Press, 1998.

———. *Sorrow's Web: Overcoming the Legacy of Maternal Depression.* New York: Free Press, 2000.

Solomon, Andrew. *The Noonday Demon: An Atlas of Depression.* New York: Scribner, 2001.

Sternberg, Esther M. *The Balance Within: The Science Connecting Health and Emotions.* New York: W. H. Freeman and Company, 2000.

Styron, William. *Darkness Visible: A Memoir of Madness.* New York: Vintage Books, 1992.

# NOTES

## Introduction

**There is no way properly to describe:** Anne Sheffield, *How You Can Survive When They're Depressed: Living and Coping with Depression Fallout* (New York: Three Rivers Press, 1999), p. viii.

## Chapter One: The Deadly Duo: Depression and Depression Fallout

**Among them psychiatrist Peter Kramer:** Peter D. Kramer, *Should You Leave?* (New York: Penguin Books, 1999), p. 160; **antidepressants work their miracle:** The Agency for Healthcare Research, Report No. 7, "Evidenced-Based Medicine," available online at www.ahcpr.gov/research/apr00.

## Chapter Two: Unraveling the Mind-Brain Mysteries of Depression

**a "need to register":** William Styron, *Darkness Visible: A Memoir of Madness* (New York: Vintage Books, 1992), p. 36; **"usurped by a noun":** *Ibid.*, p. 36; **a biological illness so serious:** "Depression Research at the National Institute of Mental Health," available online at www.nimh.nih.gov/publicat/depresfact.htm, see also, "World Health Report 2001," available online at www.who.int/-

whr/2001/main/en/chapter2/002d.htm; **and the American Medical Association:** *NAMI News,* July 1, 1999; **In 1997 its annual cost:** Robert Hirschfeld, et al., "The National Depressive and Manic-Depressive Association Consensus Statement on the Undertreatment of Depression," *Journal of the American Medical Association (JAMA)* 277, no. 4 (1997): 335; **Some 15 percent:** Kay Redfield Jamison, "Suicide and Manic-Depressive Illness," *Lifesavers,* American Suicide Foundation Newsletter, Summer, 1994; **Scientists now agree:** "Childhood Abuse and Adult Stress," *New York Times,* August 2, 2000; **Another trigger fast gaining:** Jerrold Rosenbaum, M.D., "Antidepressant Treatment and the Biology of Depression," available online at www.medscape.com; **Some researchers tie the rising prevalence:** "Dialogues on the Brain," *Harvard Mahoney Neuroscience Institute Newsletter* 2, September 28, 1993; **One of the few facts:** E. McGrath, G. P. Keita, B. R. Strickland, and N. F. Russo, eds., *National Task Force on Women and Depression: Risk Factors and Treatment* (Washington, D.C.: American Psychological Association, 1990), p. 1; **But this is open to controversy:** Jean Endicott, "Gender Similarities and Differences in the Course of Depression," *The Journal of Gender-Specific Medicine* 1:3 (1998): 40–43; **When one researcher took a hard look:** J. P. Newman, "Gender, Life Strains, and Depression: Clinical Disorder or Normal Distress?" *Journal of Health and Social Behavior* 27: 161–78; **Recently, some depression epidemiologists:** For a discussion of men and depression, and research sources, see Terrence Real, *I Don't Want to Talk About It: Overcoming the Secret Legacy of Male Depression* (New York: Scribner, 1997), pp. 22–24, 341; **Diane Spangler, a clinical psychologist:** Diane Spangler, "Study Says Men and Women Are Not Worlds Apart," *Brigham Young Magazine,* Spring, 1998; **which afflicts**

**about 2.3 million:** from the National Institute of Mental Health Web site, www.nimh.nih.publicat/manic/cfm; **"I felt a kind of numbness":** William Styron, *Darkness Visible: A Memoir of Madness,* p. 43; **"part of the psyche's":** *Ibid.,* p. 44; **"lamentable near disappearance":** *Ibid.,* p. 48; **"the sense of being accompanied":** *Ibid.,* p. 64; **"At first, everything seemed":** Kay Redfield Jamison, *An Unquiet Mind* (New York: Alfred A. Knopf, 1995), p. 36; **"My mind seemed clear":** *Ibid.,* p. 36; **her insights into:** *Ibid.,* p. 37; **"gray, bleak preoccupation with death":** *Ibid.,* p. 38.

## Chapter Three: Overcoming Denial: The Art of Persuasion

**Investigative reporters dug up:** "Tipper's Dance," *New York Times Magazine,* October 1, 2000, p. 30; **reported Ronald Reagan's:** Frank Rich, "The Last Taboo," *New York Times,* December 23, 1997; **An earlier horror story:** *Ibid*; **who both have a close relative:** *Ibid*; **One glimmer of hope:** *Ibid*; **Margot Kidder's public breakdown:** Frank Rich, "Over the Cuckoo's Nest," *New York Times,* May 4, 1996; **the ten billion spent annually:** IMS Health, available online at www.imshealth.com/public/structure/nava-content/1,3272,1034-1034-0,00.html; **I leafed through a copy:** Robert B. Cialdini, "The Science of Persuasion," *Scientific American,* February 2001, pp. 76–81.

## Chapter Four: Drawing a Line in the Sand

**Neurobiologist Oliver Sacks has observed:** Oliver Sacks, *An Anthropologist on Mars* (New York: Vintage, 1996), p. 77; **"Instead of the normal fluctuations":** Richard O'Connor, *Undoing Depression* (New York: Berkley Books, 1999), p. 103; **"Something happens that makes us angry":** *Ibid.,* p. 103; **"We know how to":** *Ibid.,* p. 4;

His description of our sense: *Ibid.*, p. 110; **"Giving in to the anger"**: *Ibid.*, p. 112; **recounts a serious falling-out:** Andrew Solomon, *The Noonday Demon* (New York: Scribner, 2001), p. 179.

## Chapter Five: A Partnership Approach to Treatment

**Ancient Greeks suffering from:** Andrew Solomon, *The Noonday Demon,* p. 286; **In nineteenth-century England:** Stephen Trombley, *All That Summer She Was Mad* (New York: Continuum, 1981), p. 157; **In 1867, an English physician:** *London Times,* March 17, 1999; **While no information is given:** National Depressive and Manic-Depressive Association, "Landmark Study Shows Gap in Patient/Physician Communication Hinders Recovery for Those with Major Depression," January 22, 2001 press release; **Most frequently prescribed are:** presentation by Joan E. Gadsby to the World Assembly for Mental Health, July 2001, available online at www.benzo.org.uk/warnh.htm; **Atypical depression, which confusingly:** "Diagnosis and Treatment of Depression," interview with Donald F. Klein, available online at www.bestdoctors.com/en/conditions/d/depression/depression_-051900_p.htm; **Although used extensively in Europe:** *Ibid*; **It is an uncomfortable truth that:** "Prescriptions: How Your Doctor Makes the Choice," *U.S. News & World Report,* February 19, 2001, pp. 58–60; **The product ads that now turn up:** "Psychiatric Drugs Are Now Promoted Directly to Patients," *New York Times,* February 17, 1998; **going off Paxil appears to create:** "Glaxo Lawsuit Could Snowball," reported September 6, 2001 on www.psychiatry.medscape.com/reuters; **the actual shock administered:** Andrew Solomon, *The Noonday Demon,* p. 121; **a list of specific recommendations:** available from the National

Depressive and Manic-Depressive Association and can be ordered online at www.ndmda.org; **news of which is accumulating:** "Herb May Weaken Birth Control," *USA Today,* May 1, 2000, and "St. John's Wort Interaction with Digozin," Editor's Correspondence, *Archives of Internal Medicine* 160 (16), September 11, 2000; **as a journalist at the** *Los Angeles Times:* "Remedy's U.S. Sales Zoom, but Quality Control Lags," *Los Angeles Times,* August 31, 1998; **has been reported as helpful:** "New Research Supports SAM-E's Potential Role in Depression Treatment," March 26, 2001, available online at www.psychiatry.medscape.com/reuters/prof/2001/03/03.26/20010323clin003.html; **A full-page** *New York Times* **advertisement:** *New York Times,* July 7, 1999; **the book's author:** author interview with Richard Brown, January 20, 2000; **Research indicates that a program:** "Aerobic Exercise Lifts Depression in Treatment-Resistant Patients," available online at www.psychiatry.medscape.com/reuters/prof/2001/04/04.06/20010405clin002.html; **In the opinion of one psychiatrist:** author interview with Donald F. Klein, February 22, 2000; **there are no less than:** "Where Does Research on the Effectiveness of Psychotherapy Stand Today?" *Harvard Mental Health Letter,* September 1995, p. 8; **One practitioner, when asked:** author interview with John Jacobs, November 13, 2001.

## Chapter Six: The Virtues of Being Selfish

**on a Broadway stage in** *Guys and Dolls:* "Adelaide's Lament," from *Guys and Dolls,* lyrics by Frank Loesser, quoted by Esther M. Sternberg in *The Balance Within* (New York: W. H. Freeman and Company, 2000), p. 11; **a wide range of physical illnesses:** Kenneth Pelletier, "Between Mind and Body: Stress, Emotions, and Health," *Mind/Body Medicine*, Daniel Goleman and Joel Gurin, eds. (Yonkers, New York: Consumer Reports Books, 1998), p. 20; **Not long ago scientists:** Esther M. Sternberg, *The Balance Within*, p. 84; **a dizzyingly complex communication system:** *Ibid.*, p. 89; **When the stressful experience:** *Ibid.*, pp. 109–10; **If, however, the stressor is prolonged:** *Ibid.*, pp. 111–12; **utilizes the central nervous system:** *Ibid.*, pp. 104–7; **Further research since then:** *Ibid.*, p. 173; **careful scientists are unwilling:** author interview with Esther M. Sternberg, March 1, 2002; **may have indulged in:** K. R. Merikangas, "Divorce and Assortative Mating Among Depressed Patients," *American Journal of Psychiatry* 141:1 (1984): 74–76; **It is, Martin writes:** Paul Martin, *The Healing Mind: The Vital Links Between Brain and Behavior, Immunity and Disease* (New York: St. Martin's Griffin, 1997), pp. 118–19; **"Those of us whose world view":** *Ibid.*, p. 123, **One pair of PNI researchers:** *Ibid.*, p. 152; **In Coyne's write-up of the experiment:** J. Kahn, J. C. Coyne, and G. Margolin, "Depression and Marital Disagreement: The Social Construction of Despair," *Journal of Social and Personal Relationships* 2 (1985): 447–61; **The truth is that in addition:** Paul Martin, *The Healing Mind*, pp. 245–49; **More than thirty years ago:** Herbert Benson, "The Relaxation Response," in *Mind/Body Medicine*, pp. 233–36; **has been thoroughly investigated:** see Paul Martin, *The Healing Mind*, pp. 164–72 and David Spiegel, "Social Support: How Friends, Family, and Groups Can Help," *Mind/Body Medicine*, pp. 331–43; **People who had just watched:** Daniel Goleman, *Emotional Intelligence* (New York: Bantam, 1997), p. 85; **Paul Martin recounts another:** Paul Martin, *The Healing Mind*, p. 134.

## Chapter Seven: I Love You, I Love You Not

**Psychiatrist Peter Kramer says:** Peter Kramer, *Should You Leave?* (New York: Penguin Books, 1999), p. 161; **prime examples of anhedonia:** *Ibid.*, p. 163; **sketches a first-visit scenario:** *Ibid.*, pp. 163–64; **His patient doesn't find:** *Ibid.*, p. 163; **"When you say that you need":** *Ibid.*, p. 163. **Dr. Kramer, who hates:** *Ibid.*, p. 166; **answered by a nameless entity called:** "Wife Says She Doesn't Love Me," available online at www.health.iafrica.com/psychonline/qa/relationshps/nolove270-1.htm; **William James (all but one of whose four siblings):** Kay Redfield Jamison, *Touched with Fire* (New York: Free Press, 1994), p. 207; **Samuel Johnson refers to his melancholy:** *Ibid.*, p. 231; **Robert Lowell equates his black moods:** *Ibid.*, p. 117; **Lord Byron, whose history of marriage:** *Ibid.*, p. 147; **The poet once wrote to a friend:** *Ibid.*, p. 171; **Jamison likens the poet's:** *Ibid.*, p. 150; **The Austrian composer Hugo Wolf:** *Ibid.*, p. 21; **most antidepressant medications cause sexual dysfunction:** R. C. Rosen, R. M. Lane, and M. Menza, "Effects of SSRIs on Sexual Function: A Critical Review," *Journal of Clinical Psychopharmacology* 19:1 (1999): 67–85; **At present, there are only three:** *Ibid*, see also, S. H. Kennedy, B. S. Eisfeld, S. E. Dickens, J. R. Bacchiochi, and R. M. Bagby, "Antidepressant-Induced Sexual Dysfunction During Treatment with Moclobemide, Paroxetine, Sertraline, and Venlafaxine," *Journal of Clinical Psychiatry* 61:4 (2000): 276–81; **The worst offenders are:** "Depression and Sex: Lifting Former Can Depress Latter," CBS Health Watch, July 20, 2001, available online at www.minisite.medscape.com/celexa/-dep_sex.html; **There are counteractive measures:** "Sexual Dysfunction in People Being Treated for Depression," presentation made by Dr. Troy L. Thompson at the American Psychiatric Association conference, March 2000, available online at www.psychiatry.medscape.com/medscape/CNO/2000/APA_IPS/-APA-12.html; **A group of experts assembled by:** "Restoring Intimacy: The Patient's Guide to Maintaining Relationships During Depression," published October 1999 by the National Depressive and Manic-Depressive Association, pp. 50–51.

## Chapter Eight: Mending or Breaking the Bond

**Infants of a depressed mother:** J. F. Cohn and E. Z. Tronick, "The Impact of Maternal Psychiatric Development on Infant Psychiatric Development," *Journal of Clinical Psychiatry* 59 (1998), pp. 53–60; **Other consequences show up:** Morris Green, "Maternal Depression: Bad for Children's Health," *Contemporary Pediatrics* 10 (November 1993), pp. 28–36; **In adolescents, they play out:** Constance Hammen, "The Family-Environmental Context of Depression: A Perspective on Children's Risk," in *Developmental Perspectives on Depression: Rochester Symposium on Developmental Psychopathology,* Dante Cicchetti and Sheree O. Toth, eds. (Rochester: University of Rochester Press, 1992), p. 266; **When researchers took a look at children:** Kyle D. Pruett, *Fatherneed: Why Father Care Is As Essential As Mother Care for Your Child* (New York: Free Press, 2000), p. 38.

# ACKNOWLEDGMENTS

My thanks go to my excellent editor, Gail Winston, for sharpening my writing and curbing my penchant for lengthy asides and extended metaphors, and to my agent, Anne Edelstein, for her unflagging support and encouragement. I am grateful as well to Richard O'Connor, Peter Jensen, Neal Aponte, and John Jacobs for answering tough questions and generously sharing their professional expertise and insights.

But my greatest debt is to the Message Board posters, whose experiences inform every page of this book and whose honesty, courage, resilience, and willingness to share their pain have bolstered my faith in the human spirit. The posters are anonymous in name only. While I have, in some instances, altered details that could compromise their real-life identities, I have used their own words to convey the stressful dynamics of relationships touched by depression and the emotional turmoil to which both partners are subject. I hope one day to offer face-to-face my thanks to Gwen, Purple, Just Me, Phil, Ginger, Windswept, and all the other depression fallout sufferers who have made this book possible. My admiration for you is boundless.

# INDEX